Books by Steven M. Fiser MD

The
ABSITE
Review

The *practice* ABSITE
Question
Book

The
Senior ABSITE
Review

The
ABS General Surgery
Oral Certifying Exam
Review
(Available 2007)

The Senior ABSITE Review
(Author of The ABSITE Review)

Steven M. Fiser MD
Hancock Surgical Consultants, LLC
Boston, Massachusetts

This book is not intended for clinical use. Extreme care has been taken to ensure the accuracy of the
    information contained in this book and to devise the safest and most conservative way of practicing
    general surgery. However, the authors and publishers are not responsible for errors or omissions in
    the book itself or from any consequences from application of the information in the book and make no
    warranty, expressed or implied, with respect to the currency, completeness, or accuracy of the
    contents of the publication. Application of this information remains the professional responsibility of
    the practitioner. The specific circumstances surrounding any individual patient requires individual
    diagnosis and treatment.

Extreme care has been taken to ensure that the drug dosages herein are accurate, however illness such as
    renal failure and other disease states can affect dose. The reader should check the package insert for
    any drug being prescribed to see the current recommended indications, warnings, and precautions.

Some drugs and devices in this text have FDA clearance only for certain indications. It is the responsibility
    of the health care provider to ascertain the FDA status of any drug or device before use.

The American Board of Surgery Inc. does not sponsor nor endorses this book.

The author has never had access to the ABSITE exams used by the American Board of Surgery Inc. other
    than to take the exam. The ABSITE Exam was not systematically reviewed for the purpose of
    creating this book. No part of this book is a specific reconstruction of a question and answer found on
    the ABSITE. Personal experiences, rigorous review of general surgery textbooks and The ABSITE
    Review were the substrates for this book.

This book was specifically written with 2 goals in mind:

1. To expand and reinforce the clinical nature of topics already covered in The ABSITE Review

2. To introduce new clinical topics not previously covered

The reader can consider this a clinical supplement to, but not a substitute for, The ABSITE Review.

Contents:

Trauma

Duodenal trauma

85% of these injuries which require operation are treated w/ **debridement** and **primary closure** or **primary anastomosis**

Segmental resection w/ primary anastomosis possible w/ all portions of duodenum except **2nd portion**

Fistulas are a major source of morbidity

Diagnosing duodenal injury

CT scan - bowel wall thickening, hematoma, air, contrast leak

UGI study best

Leak → OR, No leak → conservative tx

If CT scan worrisome for injury but non-diagnostic → repeat CT in 8 hours

Paraduodenal hematomas on CT scan

Can present with small bowel obstruction 24–72 hours after injury

Dx: Get **UGI study** to r/o leak (may show "stacked coins" or "coiled spring" findings)

Tx: Conservative treatment

TPN and NGT cures 90% of these within **3 weeks**

Clamp NGT for 4 hours every 3-4 days

Check residual over 4 hours (< 250) to see if moving gastric fluid through

Repeat UGI every week until resolution and before starting oral feeding

OR if not resolved within 3 weeks → follow **paraduodenal hematoma** below

Paraduodenal hematomas in OR (also for bile or succus drainage or fat necrosis in OR)

Kocher maneuver and open **lesser sac through omentum**

Assess wall viability, pancreas, and surrounding areas

Can inject methylene blue down NGT to look for leak

If no leak → repair serosa, **omental patch**; leave **drains NGT; NPO** for 7 days; **UGI** after that

If there is a **leak or questionable wall** integrity → primary repair or primary anastomosis

Consider IOC for injuries to 2nd portion of duodenum (or fat necrosis, bile leakage not from duodenum)

Options for operative treatment of severe duodenal injuries (leak or loss of bowel wall integrity):

1) **Primary repair** or **primary anastomosis**

2) **Jejunal serosal patch**

3) **Permanent Duodenal Exclusion**

4) **Duodenal-jejunal anastomosis**

5) **Trauma Whipple** – rarely if ever indicated

Liver trauma

Damage Control Peri-hepatic packing

Used with severe hepatic bleeding

Can **pack** severe liver injuries if patient becomes unstable or severely coagulopathic in the OR while trying to stop liver bleeding

Place packs behind, below, lateral, and over the top of the liver; want to make sure and place **lots of packs**

Close abdomen w/ IV bag (the fascia will be separated by the IV bag) to prevent compartment syndrome (occurs w/ massive resuscitation) if worried

Go to the ICU

Get patient **warmed (35-37°C)**
Fluid resuscitation with blood and coagulation factors
Blood warmer
Heating lamps
Correct coagulation studies and platelets

Go back to the OR the next day

Remove the packs
May need to keep the abdomen open for awhile

Pancreatic trauma

Suspicious fluid around pancreas on CT scan:

ERCP (or MRCP) to look for duct leak

If ERCP not available **re-CT scan** in 8 hours to see if the finding is getting worse

Follow clinical exam over that time period

Indications for OR:

Duct leak on ERCP (or MRCP)
Worsening clinical exam
Worsening finding on repeat abd CT

Kocher maneuver and open **lesser sac through omentum** to evaluate pancreas

Need to evaluate **duodenum** w/ pancreatic injuries

OR findings suspicious of pancreatic injury:

1) **Edema**
2) **Hematoma** (open these up for both penetrating and blunt)
3) **Fluid**
4) **Fat necrosis**

Primary concern is to figure out if duct involved

If duct not involved → just leave **drains**

If duct involved →

Distal pancreatic duct injury

Distal pancreatectomy (can take up to 80% of gland)

Go through the lesser sac

Usually perform **splenectomy** w/ trauma distal
pancreatectomy

Splenic vein is directly posterior to pancreas

Splenic artery is superior and posterior

Pancreatic head duct injury

Place drains initially, **delayed Whipple**
(mortality too high w/ trauma Whipple)

Whipple vs. distal pancreatectomy

Based on duct injury in relation to **SMV**

Intra-op methods for assessing whether or not the duct is injured:

1) **Look** for leaking duct

2) Intra-op **ERCP**

3) **Intra-op cholangiogram** (IOC) through gall bladder
(hope for **retrograde filling**)

MSO4 to contract sphincter of Oddi w/ this

4) Can also **transect tail of pancreas** and inject there

5) Can also **open the duodenum** and inject directly into the
ampulla of Vater

Persistent abdominal pain (or persistent amylase elevation) **following trauma**

May indicate missed (delayed) pancreatic injury

CT scans poor at diagnosing pancreatic injuries initially

Delayed signs – fluid, edema, necrosis around the pancreas

Dx: **ERCP** good at picking up delayed duct injuries

Tx: **Duct injury** → go to OR

If ERCP (and MRCP) not available → exploratory laparotomy

Following a trauma splenectomy, part of the tail of the pancreas and be inadvertently transected

Following this a pancreatic fluid collection (pancreatic fistula) can form

Usual treatment is just percutaneous drainage

ERCP w/ temporary stent if the drainage does not go down after 6 weeks

Vascular trauma

Major (hard) signs of a vascular injury:

Active hemorrhage
Pulse deficit
Expanding or pulsatile hematoma
Distal ischemia
Bruit or thrill

Tx: go to the OR emergently for exploration

1. Repair w/:

   Primary repair (< 2 cm missing) or;

   Vein interposition graft (> 2 cm missing)

2. After revascularization:

   Feel for pulse to make sure you got it back

   Feel calfs and consider prophylactic **fasciotomy** for ischemia > 4-6 hours

   Patients may present w/ ↓ pulse on that side or a tense extremity after the procedure

   Check urine myoglobin

   Check K and H → watch for washout electrolyte problems and hypotension

3. ASA post-op

Moderate (soft) signs of a vascular injury:

History of hemorrhage at the scene
Deficit in an anatomically related nerve
Large stable and non-pulsatile hematoma is present
Injury close to a major artery (i.e. GSW to the medial thigh
      or to the medial arm could potentially injure the femoral
      and axillary vessels, respectively)
ABI < 0.9
Unequal pulses

Dx: Any of above, **go to angio**

Vein injuries that require repair include:

Femoral
Popliteal
Brachiocephalic
Subclavian
Axillary

Compartment syndrome

Sx: Pain w/ passive motion; tightness

This is a clinical diagnosis, and if you highly suspect it, you should perform the fasciotomies

If your not sure, check **compartment pressures** (>20 mmHg is considered elevated)

Can occur in the upper or lower extremities

Most commonly occurs after:

Supracondylar humeral fractures
Tibial fractures
Crush injuries
Other injuries that result in a disruption and then restoration of blood flow

Undiagnosed (i.e. an intubated or unconscious patient who cannot complain of leg pain) compartment syndrome can present as:

Renal failure (from myoglobin release)

Hyperkalemia (myonecrosis and release of K)

13

Inferior Vena Cava

Cattel maneuver for exposure of the IVC (mobilizes the right colon and duodenum)

Bleeding of IVC best controlled with proximal and distal **pressure,** not clamps (can tear it)

Can place vessel loops for control

Primary repair allowed if the residual stenosis is <50% the diameter of IVC

If stenosis is > 50% of the diameter of the SVC, place saphenous vein or synthetic patch

Posterior wall IVC injuries can be repaired by cutting through the anterior wall to get exposure

Infra-renal IVC ligation

Can be performed if necessary w/ little morbidity
Consider lower extremity **fasciotomy** w/ this move

Supra-renal IVC ligation (below hepatic veins)

Will result in renal failure
Consider returning to the OR if the patient stabilizes enough post-op to allow for IVC reconstruction

Superior Mesenteric Vein

Ligation of the SMV is associated with a 10% mortality

Portal vein

Ligation of the portal vein is associated with a 50% mortality

Vertebral artery

Hemorrhage, pseudoaneurysm, or AV fistula (can hear a
continual bruit)

Tx: Go to angiography for embolization

Dissection (needs to be just vertebral; not aortic dissection)

Tx: anti-coagulation with heparin and coumadin to
prevent thrombus formation

Thrombosis

Tx: anti-coagulation with heparin and coumadin to
prevent thrombus extension

Carotid artery

Hemorrhage, pseudoaneurysm, or AV fistula (can hear a
continual bruit)

Tx: operate and primary repair or interposition graft

Dissection (needs to be just carotid; not aortic dissection)

Tx: anti-coagulate to prevent thrombus formation

Thrombosis

If antegrade flow is still present

Tx: operate and primary repair or interposition graft

Without antegrade flow

Tx: anti-coagulate to prevent thrombus extension

Extremity Vascular Injuries

Small intimal flaps, small segmental stenoses, small pseudoaneurysms, AVF's, small focal narrowings, and dissections - all of which are <u>not</u> flow limiting:

Tx: heparin, transitioned to coumadin

Careful F/U during admission and after discharge w/ duplex studies

If there is any doubt, just operate

If there is flow limitation

Tx: operate and primary repair or interposition graft

Glasgow Coma Scale (GCS)

Motor Function

6 follows commands
5 localizes to the pain site
4 withdrawals from the pain
3 flexion with painful stimuli (decorticate)
2 extension with painful stimuli (decerebrate)
1 no response to painful stimuli

Verbal Response

5 oriented x 3
4 confused but responds
3 inappropriate words with speech
2 incomprehensible sounds (grunting)
1 no response verbally

Eye opening

4 spontaneous eye opening
3 opens eyes to command
2 opens eyes to pain
1 no response to eye opening

Best prognostic indicator of GCS is the motor component.

Larynx and Trachea Trauma

Are considered to be **airway emergencies**

Sx: crepitus in the neck

Respiratory stridor

Respiratory compromise

Hoarseness

Secure the airway emergently in ER

Awake fiberoptic intubation if the patient is still breathing

Awake cricothyroidotomy or tracheostomy if can't get
fiberoptic

Perform these procedures with only local anesthetics so
the patient can maintain his airway

After securing the airway, go to OR for repair of injury

Usually just perform primary repair of the injury

Tracheosotmy (7.5 cuffed Shiley for adult) is placed

Protects airway from edema which secondary to trauma

Allows easy method of checking for stricture at repair site

If you have performed a cricothyroidotomy:

Need conversion to tracheostomy in first 7 days or so to
prevent voice problems and scarring of the larynx

Ureteral trauma

Single shot intravenous pyelogram (IVP)

Consider this with penetrating wounds to the lower abdominal quadrants (or if worried about ureteral injury for some other reason)

This will identify injury and presence of 2 functional kidney's

Ureteral injuries above the pelvic brim (upper and middle third injuries)

If large segment is missing (>2 cm)

Likely will <u>not</u> reach bladder w/ a bladder hitch

Need to temporize with **percutaneous nephrostomy**

Tie off both ends of the ureter

Can go with **ileal interposition** or **trans-ureteroureterostomy** later

If small segment is missing (< 2 cm)

Spatulate ends and perform **primary repair** (6-0 PDS sutures)

Repair over a stent

Ureteral injuries below the pelvic brim (lower third injuries)

All of these injuries are re-implanted in the bladder if a segment is missing

5-0 monocryl for ureteral to bladder mucosa anastomosis

Fold **bladder muscle** over ureter so you don't get **vesico-ureteral reflux**

May need **bladder (psoas) hitch** procedure to get the ureter to reach

Need to avoid stripping the ureters in order to preserve blood supply

Intravenous indigo carmine or methylene blue can be used to find injuries or check for leaks after repair

Leave drains for all ureteral injuries

Renal trauma

Hematuria best indicator of renal trauma

95% of injuries are treated **non-operatively**

Not all urine extravasation requires operation

All patients with hematuria will need a **CT scan**

Indications for operation w/ blunt renal trauma:

Acute phase

Ongoing hemorrhage w/ instability

After acute phase

Major collecting system disruption
Unresolving urine extravasation
Severe hematuria

Intravenous methylene blue (1 mg/kg) - can be used to find leak intra-op

Anterior to posterior renal hilum structures – **renal vein, renal artery, renal pelvis (VAP)**

Left renal vein

Can ligate near IVC (has **adrenal vein** and **gonadal vein** collaterals)

Right does <u>not</u>

With exploration try to get control of **vascular hilum 1st**

Left side → Mattox

Right side → Cattel

Dissect through **Gerota's fascia**, get proximal and distal control

Expanding peri-renal hematomas → open

> If considering nephrectomy, IVP to confirm contra-lateral kidney

Non-expanding peri-renal hematomas → Get IVP

> If vascular injury, open and repair, o/w leave it alone

Can use SVG if not enough length for renal artery or renal vein repair

Place **drains**, especially if collecting system is injured

IV Methylene blue dye injection can be used at the end of the case to check for leak (as above)

Orthopaedic Trauma

Long bone fractures or dislocations with a loss of pulse (or weak pulse)

Perform immediate reduction of the fracture or dislocation and see if the pulse returns:

Pulse does not return after reduction

Tx: operate and primary repair or interposition graft

Make incision at the site of the fracture or the dislocation

Can get and intra-op angiogram if not sure of the location of the injury

If the patient's pulse is weak or the ABI < 0.9

Tx: angiogram to see if there is an injury

Can have over a **2 L blood loss** from a femur fracture

Knee dislocations

Pulse is absent after reduction:

Tx: operate and primary repair or interposition graft

Posterior approach to popliteal artery w/ trauma

Pulse is present after reduction:

Tx: angiography (all patients with knee dislocations automatically get an angiogram because of the high incidence of popliteal artery injury)

23

Upper Extremity Injury	**Nerve or Artery Trauma**
Anterior shoulder dislocation	**Axillary Nerve**
Posterior shoulder dislocation	**Axillary Artery**
Proximal humerus fracture	**Axillary Nerve**
Middle humerus fracture (also a spiral humerus fracture)	**Radial Nerve**
Distal humerus fracture (also a supra-condylar humerus fracture)	**Brachial Artery**
Elbow dislocation	**Brachial Artery**
Distal radius fracture	**Median Nerve**

Lower Extremity Injury	**Nerve or Artery Trauma**
Anterior hip dislocation	**Femoral artery**
Posterior hip dislocation	**Sciatic nerve**
Distal femur fracture (supracondylar)	**Popliteal artery**
Posterior knee dislocation	**Popliteal artery**
Fibula neck fracture	**Common peroneal nerve**

24

Critical Care

Swan Ganz Catheter Normal Values (ranges) for Adults

Cardiac output (CO)	**6** (4 - 8 L/min)
Cardiac index (CI)	**3** (2.5 - 4 L/min)
Systemic vascular resistance	**1100** (800-1400 dynes)
Wedge pressure	**11** (8-14)
Central venous pressure (CVP)	**7** (5-9)
Pulmonary artery pressure	25/10
Mixed venous oxygen saturation (SVO_2)	**70** (65-75)

	Wedge Pressure	CI	SVR
Hemorrhagic shock	↓	↓	↑
Septic (hyperdynamic) shock	↓ (most commonly)*	↑*	↓
Cardiogenic shock	↑	↓	↑
Neurogenic shock	↓	↓	↓
Hypoadrenal shock	↓ (most commonly)**	↓	↓

*Patients with late septic shock can present with an elevated wedge pressure and lowered CI as the heart starts to give out

**Patients with hypoadrenal shock can present with an elevated wedge pressure although this would not be the classic finding

Diabetics have increased SVR

Primary determinants of myocardial oxygen consumption

   Wall tension (most important)
   Heart rate

Inotropes

   Milrinone
   Dobutamine
   Dopamine (Medium to high dose)
   Amrinone
   Epinephrine (also a pressor)

Pressors

   Norepinephrine
   Phenylephrine

Mechanism of various inotropes

   Inotropes that directly increase cAMP

      Norepinephrine (mostly a pressor, some inotropic activity)
      Epinephrine (mostly an inotrope, some pressor activity)
      Dopamine
      Dobutamine

   Inotropes that inhibit cAMP phosphodiesterase (indirectly
      increased cAMP)

      Milrinone

   Inotropes that inhibit Na/K transporter

      Digoxin

Mechanism of various pressors

Phenylephrine – pure alpha agonist

Norepinephrine – beta and alpha agonist

Various Deficiencies and Side-Effects

Trace elements   Can lead to poor wound healing

Thiamine (B_1)   Wernicke's encephalopathy
Cardiomyopathy (wet beri-beri)
Peripheral neuropathy, lateral gaze palsy
Cerebellar ataxia

Pyridoxine (B_6)
Deficiency   Sideroblastic anemia
Glossitis
Peripheral neuropathy

Cobalamin (B_{12})
Deficiency   Megaloblastic anemia
Glossitis
Peripheral neuropathy

Folate Deficiency   Megaloblastic anemia
Glossitis
NO peripheral neuropathy

Niacin Deficiency   Pellagra
    Diarrhea
    Dermatitis
    Dementia

Phosphate
deficiency   Generalized weakness
Failure to wean from the ventilator
Encephalopathy
Decreased macrophage phagocytosis

Vitamin A
Deficiency   Can cause night blindness

Vitamin K
Deficiency   Can result in coagulopathy (elevated PT)

Vitamin D Deficiency	Ricketts in children Osteomalacia in adults
Vitamin E Deficiency	Peripheral neuropathy (can occur w/ fat malabsorption)

Electrolyte Disorders

Sodium

Normal value: 135-145

Hypernatremia

Tx: Correct slowly w/ 1/2 NS to avoid **brain swelling**
Want sodium to be corrected at 1 mEq/hr

Free water deficit = 0.6 x wt. (kg) x [(serum Na/140) – 1]

Hyponatremia

Tx: **1st water restriction** (first line therapy)
2nd diuresis
3rd NaCl replacement

Correct Na slow to avoid **central pontine myelinosis**

Sodium deficit = 0.6 x wt. (kg) x (140 – Na)

Pseudohyponatremia

Elevated glucose levels can lower sodium levels artificially

For each 100 increment of glucose over 100, add 2 to the sodium value

Pseudohyponatremia can also occur with hyper-triglyeridemia (can occur with pancreatitis)

Potassium

Normal Value: 3.5 – 5.0

Hyperkalemia

EKG - peaked T waves, QRS will start to widen

Tx: 1 amp calcium gluconate (membrane stabilizer for heart)

1 amp sodium bicarbonate (causes alkalosis, K enters cell in exchange for H)

10 U insulin and 1 ampule of 50% dextrose (K driven into cells along with glucose)

Kaexylate

Albuterol Nebs

Lasix

Dialysis if refractory

Hypokalemia

EKG - T waves disappear

Tx: potassium

Calcium

Normal value: 8.5 – 10.5

Hypercalcemia (symptoms usually occur at > 13)

Sx: Lethargy
Decreased tendon reflexes
Shortened QT interval

Breast cancer MC malignant cause

Tx:
Normal saline, 200-300 cc/hr
<u>No</u> lactated ringers – contains Ca

Lasix
<u>No</u> thiazide diuretics – reabsorb Ca

Malignant disease
Mithramycin
Calcitonin
Aldaronic acid

Hypocalcemia (symptoms usually occur at < 8)

Sx: Hyperreflexes
Chvostek's sign (tapping on face produces twitching)
Perioral tingling and numbness
Trousseau's sign (carpopedal spasm)
Prolonged QT interval

Tx: **Calcium**
May need to **correct Mg** before able to correct Ca

Magnesium

Normal value: 2.0 - 2.7

Hypermagnesemia

Sx: Lethargy (symptoms similar to hypercalcemia)
Usually occurs with burns, trauma or renal dialysis

Tx: **calcium**
Hemodialysis

Hypomagnesemia

Sx: Symptoms similar to hypocalcemia
Hyperreflexes
Chvostek's sign
Perioral tingling and numbness
Trousseau's sign

Tx: Magnesium

Hemodialysis can remove elevated **K, Ca, PO4,** and **Mg**

Total Peripheral Nutrition (TPN)

Calculating TPN

Protein: 1 gm **protein**/kg/day (20% essential amino acids)

Fat: 50% of non-protein calories **fat**

Dextrose: 50% of non-protein calories **dextrose**

Additional components that must be added:

Trace elements (Zn, Cu, Mg, Cr)

Vitamins (usually comes in mixture)
Vit K not included and needs to be added separately

Electrolytes (**Na** – 2 mEq/kg/day, **K** – 1 mEq/kg/day, Ca, Mg, Cl, PHO4, and acetate)

Better to use the gastrointestinal tract if at all possible (prevents bacterial translocation)

Short term TPN complicated by issues associated with indwelling catheters (line sepsis, pneumothorax, etc.)

Long term TPN can eventually lead to cirrhosis

Starvation or Major Stress (Surgery, Trauma, Systemic Illness)

Glycogen

Stored in skeletal muscle (2/3) and liver (1/3)

Glycogen stores are depleted after 24–36 hours of starvation

Body starts breaking down **fat stores** when glycogen runs out

Skeletal muscle is deficient in **glucose-6 phosphatase**

> This enzyme is only found in **liver**

> Because of this deficiency, glucose-6 phosphate stays in muscle after glycogen breakdown and is utilized there.

Gluconeogenesis

Precursors

Amino acids (especially alanine)
Lactic acid
Acetate
Pyruvate
Glycerol

Alanine is simplest and primary substrate for gluconeogenesis

> **Alanine** and **phenylalanine** are the only amino acids to increase during trauma, starvation, stress

Liver – primary site of gluconeogenesis

Kidney – gluconeogenesis occurs here **late in starvation**

Trauma

Protein-sparing does <u>not</u> occur with **trauma**

High levels of **catecholamines and cortisol** prevent protein conservation

Starvation

Protein-sparing occurs with **starvation**

Toxicities

Nipride

Can cause **cyanide toxicity**

Cyanide binds to cytochrome c in mitochondria and disrupts the electron transport chain

Cell cannot use oxygen so you get a left to right shunt

Tx: amyl nitrite, then sodium nitrite

Carbon monoxide

Causes – fire with inhalation of gases

Increases affinity of Hgb for oxygen (left shift)

Hard to release oxygen to the tissues

Abnormal levels of carboxyhemoglobin

Normal patients >10%

Smokers >20%

Tx: 100% oxygen on ventilator (displaces carbon monoxide).

Can also use hyperbaric O_2

Methemoglobinemia

Causes – nitrites such as hurricaine spray, fertilizers, fungicides

Prevents O2 binding to Hgb (right shift)

Tx: methylene blue
vitamin C

Renal Failure

Hypotension – most common cause of postoperative renal failure

$$FeNa = \frac{(urine\ Na/Cr)}{(plasma\ Na/Cr)}$$

Pre-renal renal failure

FeNa <1%
Urine Na <20
BUN/Cr ratio >20
Urine osmolality >500 mOsm

Oliguria

1st – volume resuscitation (CVP 15)
2nd –diuretics to try and convert to non-oliguric renal failure
3rd – dialysis for volume overload, electrolyte disorders, etc
(see below)

Electrolyte abnormalities with renal failure

Volume overload
Decreased Na and Ca
Increased K, PO4, and Mg

Indications for dialysis

Fluid overload
Increased K
Metabolic acidosis
Uremic encephalopathy
Uremic coagulopathy
Poisoning

Excessive PEEP complications

↓ left atrial filling
↓ cardiac output
↓ renal blood flow
↓ urine output

↑ pulmonary vascular resistance

Effects of obesity on pulmonary function

Decreased FVC
Decreased FEV-1
Decreased FRC

Acid-base balance

	pH	CO_2	HCO_3
Respiratory acidosis	↓	↑	↑
Respiratory alkalosis	↑	↓	↓
Metabolic acidosis	↓	↓	↓
Metabolic alkalosis	↑	↑	↑

Lungs modulate pH by regulating CO_2

Kidney modulates pH by regulating H ion

Occurs at the level of the collecting system

Primarily under the influence of aldosterone

Malignant causes of hypercalcemia

Hematologic malignancies (25%)

Results in lytic bone lesions and release of Ca

Non-hematologic malignancies (75%)

Cancers that release **PTH-rp**

Includes breast CA (most common), squamous cell lung CA

Breast cancer is the most common cause of malignant hypercalcemia (due to elevated PTH-rp)

Urine cAMP will be high in malignant hypercalcemia related to PTH-rp and normal in malignant hypercalcemia related to hematologic malignancy

CO2 embolus during laparoscopic cholecystectomy

Remove CO2 insufflation

Place the patients **head down** and the patient on the **left side** (to prevent any more propagation of CO2 into the lungs)

Increase minute ventilation (RR and TV) to help reabsorb the CO2 embolus

100% oxygen is given which is absorbed faster than CO2

> The oxygen will come to equilibrium with the CO2 in the embolus and will be reabsorbed faster than the CO2

> Will also help oxygenate the patient

If CPR is needed, it should progress for a prolonged period of time to allow the embolus to be re-absorbed.

Can place central line and try to aspirate CO2

Wound Healing

Open wounds

Epithelial integrity is the most important factor in healing by secondary intention

Epithelial cells migrate from wound edges, sweat glands, and hair follicles

Need granulation tissue for epithelialization to occur

Lack of epithelialization results in leakage of serum and proteins which promotes bacteria growth

Closed Incisions

Tensile strength is the most important factor in healing by primary intention

Relies on the deposition of collagen and subsequent **cross-linking**

The strength layer of bowel is the **submucosa**

Approximately **3-5 days** is the weakest time point for small bowel anastomosis

Myofibroblasts

Cell that causes wound contraction

Combination smooth muscle–fibroblast cell

Communication through gap junctions

Steroids

Steroids inhibit macrophages, PMN's, and collagen synthesis by fibroblasts which retards wound healing

Also decreases wound tensile strength

Vitamin A - effectively prevents the negative effects of steroids on wound healing

Infection and Immunity

Common Infections

MC organism in gram negative sepsis – E Coli

MC organism in surgical wound infections – staph aureus

MC anaerobe in surgical wound infections – Bacteriodies fragilis

MC fungal infection – Candida

MC non-surgical infection – urinary tract infection

MCC of infectious death after surgery – nosocomial pneumonia

MC organism for nosocomial pneumonia – staph aureus

MC class of organism for nosocomial pneumonia – GNR's

MC organism in spontaneous bacterial peritonitis – E. Coli

MC organism in line infection – staph epidermidis

Bacteriodies Fragilis – most common anaerobe in the colon.

E. Coli – most common aerobic bacteria in the colon

Most potent stimulus of TNF release – endotoxin (lipopolysaccharide, Lipid A complex)

Occurs with gram negative sepsis

Clostridium difficile colitis

Associated with antibiotic use
Rarely can result in toxic colitis requiring colectomy
Toxin A (enterotoxin) seems to be responsible for the acute
    inflammatory response
Forms yellow to gray pseudomembranes
Dx: ELISA for Toxin A best test; fecal leukocytes
Tx: IV or PO flagyl, PO vancomycin
    IVF's rehydration
    Avoid anti-motility agents

Cytomegalovirus infection

AIDS patients
MC manifestation is **CMV colitis**
MC reason for a laparotomy in patients with AIDS is CMV
    colitis
CMV colitis can result in bowel perforation or bleeding

Transplant recipients
MC infectious agent in transplant recipients
MC manifestation is febrile mononucleosis
Can get CMV pneumonitis (most deadly form of CMV
    infection in transplant recipients)

Biopsies - show characteristic cellular inclusion bodies

Tx:
Gangciclovir
Side effects – CNS toxicity, bone marrow suppression
Usually given prophylactically in TXP patients

CMV-IVIG (CMV immunoglobulin)
Given for severe infections
Also given in transplantation for CMV negative recipient
    and CMV positive donor
Side effects – nausea, vomiting, flushing

Immunoglobulins

IgM – 1st antibody produced with infection

IgG – most abundant Ab in the body

IgA – in secretions; GI tract; breast milk

IgE – involved in allergic reactions

IgM and IgG are both opsonins and both can fix complement

Newborn Immunodeficiencies

All limbs of the immune system are impaired

PMN chemotaxis and deformability are reduced

Lower T-cell activity

Low levels of IgA, IgM, IgD, and IgE at birth (these do not cross the placenta)

IgG does cross the placenta but drops in levels shortly after birth as it is catabolized

IgA is passed to the infant through breast milk

Indications for bacterial endocarditis prophylaxis at time of surgery;

Previous valve surgery
Mitral valve prolapse with mitral regurgitation
Complex congenital heart disease
Surgical PA to systemic shunts
Previous endocarditis
Hypertrophic cardiomyopathy

Generally just give a second generation cephalosporin pre-op and for 48 hours post-op

Adoptive Immunotherapy

Harvest host T-cells

Add IL-2 to activate these cells

Forms lymphokine activate T killer cells (LAK cells)

These cells attack the tumor

Can also add a tumor antigen which will create tumor specific LAK cells

Has been used for melanoma with some success

Nutrition

Caloric need = approximately 20-25 kcal/kg/day (resting energy expenditure)

(see critical care section for calculation for TPN)

Minor surgery (i.e. laparoscopic cholecystectomy)

Increases kcal requirement (resting energy expenditure) 10%

Major surgery, trauma or sepsis

Increases kcal requirement (resting energy expenditure) 20%–40%.

Early enteral feeding

Sepsis and pancreatitis are the best indications

Reduced mortality in septic patients

Harris Benedict Equation

Calculates resting (basal) energy expenditure based on age, height, weight, and gender

Fluid replacement

Gastric losses (i.e. NG tube suctioning)

Tx: D5 ½ NS w/ 20 mEq K

High output small bowel fistula (or high output iliostomy)

Tx: lactated ringers with HCO3-

Severe Diarrhea (i.e. clostridium difficile colitis)

Tx: lactated ringers with K+

Trauma

Tx: lactated ringers initially

Pharmacology

Common Antibiotics

Ancef (1-2 gm TID)

Cefoxitin (1-2 gm TID)

Zosyn (3.375 mg QID)

Cefepime (1-2 gm IV BID)

Levofloxacin (250-500 QD)

Vancomycin (15 mg/kg BID)

Gentamicin (1mg/kg QID)

Flagyl (500 mg TID)

Assessment of peak and trough

If the trough is too high, need to decrease the frequency (increase the interval between doses)

If the peak is too high, need to decrease the dose

Immunosuppressive Drugs

Steroids

Inhibit cytokine synthesis (IL-1, IL-6)
Inhibit macrophages
Side effects – Cushing's syndrome

Cyclosporin (CSA)

Binds **cyclophilin protein**
Inhibits cytokine synthesis (IL-2, IL-3, IL-4, INF-gamma).
Undergoes hepatic metabolism and biliary excretion
Side effects - nephrotoxicity, seizures

FK-506 (Prograf)

Binds **FK binding protein**
Similar to cyclosporin, but 10–100x more potent
Side effects – nephrotoxicity, mood changes, GI problems

Azathioprine (Imuran)

Inhibits purine synthesis required by T cells
Thus, inhibits T cells
Active metabolite - 6-mercaptopurine
    Metabolite formed in the liver
Side effects
    Myelosuppression (keep wbc's > 3)
    Possible lymphoproliferative disease

Mycophenolate (MMF)

Similar action to azathioprine
Side effects (similar to azathioprine)
    Myelosuppression (keep wbc's > 3)
    Possible lymphoproliferative disease

ATGAM

51

Equine polyclonal antibodies against T cell Ag's
Used for induction
Complement dependent
Side effects - myelosuppression

Thymoglobulin

Rabbit polyclonal antibodies against T cell Ag's
Similar to ATGAM
Used for induction
Side effects - myelosuppression

OKT3

Monoclonal antibodies which bind CD3
Block antigen recognition function of T cells
Results in complement dependent opsonization of T cells
Indicated for severe rejection episodes
Can have significant side effects: fever, rigors, chills, severe
pulmonary edema, and shock

Zenepax

Monoclonal antibody to IL-2 receptors (human)
Indicated for induction and rejection episodes

Rapamycin

Mechanism is by binding the FK binding protein but then
binds a separate target called the mTOR (mammalian
target of rapamycin)

The Rapamycin-FKBP-mTOR complex inhibits the pathways
involved in cell cycle progression

Infliximab (remicade)

Ab to TNF-alpha

Used for Crohn's disease, especially for the treatment of fistulas
(primary indication)

Contraindications

Allergy to rodents
Active infections
CHF

Increased risk of malignancy with Infliximab

Especially lymphoma
Risk may be further increased by other immunosuppressive
medication such as Imuran

Burns

Wash off and clean burns (warm water/soap)

Silvadene over area, telfa, wrap loosely w/ gauze

Sulfamylon for cartilagenous areas

Tetanus shot

1st **week** – excise **burned areas** and start **nutrition**

> **Early excision of burned areas** (48-72 hours after burn)
>
> > Use dermatome for deep 2nd degree and 3rd degree wound
> >
> > > Viability of skin after excision is based on:
> > >
> > > > **Color**
> > > > **Texture**
> > > > **Punctate bleeding** after removal
> > >
> > > Thrombin or epi soaked pads to help control bleeding
> >
> > Skin grafts need to be **compressed** down w/ xeroform gauze and cotton balls
> >
> > > Prevents seroma or hematoma from forming which prevents graft from attaching
> >
> > 3-0 nylons to hold down dressing

Infected areas

Can be covered w/ allograft and re-excised later

Biopsy suspected burn wound infections

Auto-grafts contraindicated if culture positive for **bacteria >10^5**

Best Dx method for burn wound sepsis is **burn wound biopsy**

Donor site w/ xeroform

Will heal in **3 weeks** and can use as a donor site again

No allograft in **pregnant women**

Reported fetal deaths from HLA mismatch

FTSG can be harvested from **behind ear**, just **above clavicle**, or **groin**

Need to have **periosteum** intact if contemplating a skin graft to bone

Limits for each burn wound excision session:

< 1 liter blood loss
< 20% of burn excised
< 2 hours total in the OR
Blood loss is to be expected
Can get extremely sick w/ too much OR time

Skin graft loss

MC due to seroma or hematoma formation under graft

2nd week – specialized areas are now addressed, allograft replaced with autograft

Face – topical antibiotics for 1 week, full-thickness grafts for unhealed areas (non-meshed)

Hands - immobilize in functional position and abx's for 1 week

Then graft (FTSG) and immobilize in functional position for 1 week after operation

Then physical therapy

May need wire fixation of joints if unstable or open

Genitals – topical abx's for 1 week. Graft unhealed areas. Can use meshed.

Transplantation

Kidney transplantation

Kidney Evaluation for suspected Acute Rejection

Increased creatnine or a decrease in urine output usually initiates evaluation for rejection

Duplex Ultrasound:

Check for vascular stricture, compression, or thrombosis

Check for ureteral obstruction or other fluid collections which may suggest a urine leak

Biopsy the kidney

Acute Kidney Rejection

Most commonly occurs within the 1st 6 months

Pathology shows

Tubulitis (mild to moderate rejection)
Vasculitis (severe rejection)

Tx: pulse steroids (500 mg of solumedrol typical)

May increase cyclosporin or prograf

OKT3, thymoglobulin, ATGAM, and zenepax can be used for severe episodes

Chronic Kidney Rejection

Unusual for this to occur < 1 year after transplantation

No effective treatment

Liver transplantation

Cholangitis

PMN's surrounding the portal triad

Do not see mixed infiltrate as you would with rejection

Liver Evaluation for suspected Acute Rejection

Symptoms of acute rejection

Fever
Jaundice
Decreased bile output
Change in bile consistency

Labs may show

Leukocytosis
Eosinophilia
Increased LFTs (total bilirubin)
Increased PT

Need to get **liver biopsy**

Acute Liver Rejection

Most commonly occurs in the 1st 2 months

Pathology shows:

Portal lymphocytosis
Endothelitis (mixed infiltrate)
Bile duct injury

Tx: pulse steroids (500 mg of solumedrol typical)

May increase cyclosporin or prograf

OKT3, thymoglobulin, ATGAM, and zenepax can be
used for severe episodes

Chronic Liver Rejection

Bile ducts start disappearing

Both antibody and cellular attack on bile ducts occurs

Gradual bile duct obstruction

Alkaline phosphatase increases

Portal fibrosis

Acute rejection is the most common predictor for chronic
rejection

No real effective treatment

Plastics, Skin, and Soft Tissue

Melanoma

Treatment of the primary melanoma:

Melanoma in situ (Hutchinson's Freckle if on face) – 0.5 cm margins OK

Thin melanoma (< 1 mm) – 1 cm margin

Intermediate melanoma (1-4 mm) – 2 cm margin

Thick melanoma (> 4 mm) – 2-3 cm margin (based on location)

Nodal Disease Work-up:

Intermediate and thick melanomas (> 1 mm) get **SLNBx**

Exception is pt's w/ clinically positive nodes, then just perform LN dissection

Thin melanoma (< 1 mm) characteristics that indicate need for **SLNBx:**

Ulceration

Regression on pathology (was deeper at one point but regressed)

If into the **reticular dermis**

Clinically positive nodes → need formal dissection (No SLNBx)

Nodal DZ but can't find primary → formal
lymphadenectomy

Metastatic Disease w/u:

Intermediate and thick melanomas require:

Chest/Abdominal/Pelvic CT

LFT's

LDH

Thin melanoma w/ clinically positive nodes also need same
w/u

Face (head and neck) melanoma

Scalp or face anterior to ear pinna and superior to lip usually go the **parotid region**

Lesions inferior to the lip commissure go to the **anterior cervical chain**

Lesions behind the pinna of the ear go to the **posterior cervical chain**

Anterior head melanoma:

SLNBx

If parotid lights → superficial parotidectomy

Take all blue nodes and any nodes ≥ 10% of the node w/ the highest gamma count

If superficial parotid contains tumor, need total parotidectomy

Clinically positive adenopathy → MRND (level I-V nodes), include superficial parotidectomy

Positive nodes on SLNBx (requires re-operation)→ MRND (level I-V nodes), include superficial parotidectomy

Posterior head melanoma

SLNBx

Take all blue nodes and any nodes ≥ 10% of the node w/ the highest gamma count

Clinically positive adenopathy → MRND (level I-V nodes)

Positive nodes on SLNBx (requires re-operation)→ MRND (level I-V nodes)

Subungal melanoma

Remove the nail and get a punch Bx

Thumb melanoma– amputate at the DIP joint

Any other finger melanoma → amputate at the PIP

Toe melanoma→ amputate at the MTP joint

Anal canal

Make sure you have met's w/u before contemplating APR

Thin melanoma → excise to appropriate margins

Thick melanoma → APR

Intermediate melanoma → case by case basis, thicker lesions lean towards APR (Discuss w/ pt)

Foot melanoma

Need special pedicled, myofascial cutaneous flaps for the sole of the foot (plastics needs to handle this)

Systemic treatment for melanoma

Interferon
IL-2
Tumor vaccines

Melanoma is associated w/ **s-100** and **HMB-45** tumor markers

Congenital nevus

These lesions have malignant potential for melanoma (10%)

Can be quite large

Not removed prophylactically unless small (< 2 cm)

tx frequent follow-up to look for change in the nevus

If melanoma found, need to resect the whole nevus (may need rotational flap or STSG)

TRAM Flaps

Blood supply is from peri-umbilical perforators

Skin grafts

Get nutrients by **imbibition** (osmotic flow) for the 1st 48 hours

Hemangioma

Can arise at time of birth or shortly after

Usual sequence is rapid growth during the first year of life but then gradually involutes

Tx: observation usual

90% are gone by **age 5-6**

Characteristics that indicate the need for treatment of hemangiomas:

Uncontrollable growth

Impaired function

Airway
Eyelid
Ear canal

Persistent after age 8

Tx:

Systemic steroids

Intra-lesional steroids

Resection if medical therapy is unsuccessful

Can also use laser therapy

Merkel cell carcinoma

Neuroendocrine tumor of the skin

Malignant

Has aggressive regional and systemic spread

Appears as a red to purple nodule or indurated area

Features on pathology

> **neuron-specific enolase (NSE)**
> **cytokeratin**
> **neurofilament protein**

Tx: resection

Glomus cell tumor

Tumor has blood vessels and nerves

Benign

Very painful

Most commonly in the tip of a digit

Tx: tumor excision

Head and Neck

Enlarged Neck Node or Neck Mass Work up

If inflammatory, can treat w/ antibiotics w/ follow-up in 2 weeks

1st – **CXR** and **core needle** (in office, that day)

If it shows malignant cells, base w/u on type of cells

If indeterminant, follow below

2nd – **Bronchoscopy/EGD/colonoscopy**

Neck/chest/abd/pelvic CT

Mammogram in women

All of these studies focused on trying to find the primary

3rd – still not sure → **excisional biopsy**

Send FS

Need to be prepared for MRND (for thyroid CA, melanoma, or some SCCA)

Core needle Bx or excisional Bx shows:

Inflammatory cells→ Abx's, back in 2 weeks

Melanoma → need MRND

Adenocarcinoma – if breast, esophagus, or lung primary →
unresectable (chemo-XRT)

SCCA

If lung or esophagus primary → unresectable (chemo-XRT)

If ENT tumor → MRND; resect ENT tumor

Can't find any primary – MRND; then XRT to area around primary

Lymphoma

Just perform excisional Bx or core needle biopsy only (<u>no</u> formal neck dissection)

Stage w/ neck/chest/abdominal CT and Bone marrow Bx

Tx: Chemo-XRT

Thyroid CA

Follow appropriate treatment

Ludwig's Angina

Thyroid

Thyroid nodule evaluation

1st Thyroid function tests

Elevated – give thyroxin (hyper-functioning nodule)

Nodule should regress in 6 months.

If the nodule does not regress, get an FNA.

Not elevated – get an FNA

2nd Fine-needle aspiration

Determinant in 85% → follow appropriate treatment

Follicular cells → lobectomy (possible total thyroidectomy)

10% malignancy risk

Thyroid CA → lobectomy (possible total thyroidectomy)

Cyst fluid → drain fluid (send to cytology)

If it recurs → thyroidectomy or lobectomy

Papillary cystic CA can present as a cyst

Colloid tissue → likely a colloid goiter

Low malignancy risk (<1%)

Just follow these and FNA for change in
characteristics

Indeterminant in 15% → need a radionuclide study

Hot nodule

Thyroxin therapy for 6 months

Size of the lesion should start to decrease

If lesion does not regress, perform **lobectomy**

Cold nodule

Thyroidectomy or lobectomy indicated

Cold nodules are more likely to be malignant than
hot nodules

Papillary thyroid carcinoma

Pathology

> Psammoma bodies
> Orphan annie nuclei
> Most common thyroid CA associated with previous XRT

Perform **lobectomy** initially, send for FS and permanent

Indications for **total thyroidectomy:**

> **Tumor > 1 cm**
> **Extrathyroidal DZ** (capsular invasion, nodal DZ, or met's)
> **Multicentric DZ**
> Hx of **XRT**

Indications for **MRND:**

> **Extrathyroidal DZ** (capsule invasion, nodal DZ or mets)

Indications for ^{131}I (6 weeks after surgery):

> **Tumor > 1cm**
> **Extrathyroidal DZ** (capsule invasion, nodal DZ or mets)

No thyroid replacement after resection until after treatment w/ ^{131}I

> Keeps TSH high (3 x normal) for ^{131}I
> Want to avoid suppressing ^{131}I uptake

After tx w/ ^{131}I, **give synthroid** to keep TSH levels low

> Want TSH ≤ 0.03 and pt mildly thyrotoxic
> This is very effective tx for any residual DZ

XRT only for unresectable DZ not responsive to ^{131}I

Can follow **thyroglobulin** post-op for tumor recurrence (if you
have done a total thyroidectomy)

Metastases go to **lung** (rare)

5-year survival – 95%

71

Follicular thyroid carcinoma

Perform **lobectomy** initially, send for FS and permanent

Indications for **total thyroidectomy:**

> **Tumor > 1 cm**
> **Extrathyroidal DZ** (capsular invasion, nodal DZ, or met's)
> **Multicentric DZ**
> Hx of **XRT**

Indications for **MRND:**

> **Extrathyroidal DZ** (capsule invasion, nodal DZ or mets)

Indications for ^{131}I (6 weeks after surgery):

> **Tumor > 1cm**
> **Extrathyroidal DZ** (capsule invasion, nodal DZ or mets)

No thyroid replacement after resection until after treatment w/ ^{131}I

> Want to avoid suppressing ^{131}I uptake
> Keeps TSH high (3 x normal) for ^{131}I

After tx w/ ^{131}I, **give synthroid** to keep TSH levels low

> Want TSH $\leq$ 0.03 and pt mildly thyrotoxic
> This is very effective tx for any residual DZ

XRT only for unresectable DZ not responsive to ^{131}I

Can follow **thyroglobulin** post-op for tumor recurrence (if you have done a total thyroidectomy)

Metastases go to **bone**

5-year survival -70%

Risk factors for metastatic spread and/or recurrence w/ papillary and follicular thyroid CA (AMES plus XRT)

Previous XRT

Age < 20 or > 50

Males

Extra-capsular invasion

Size > 1 cm

Medullary thyroid carcinoma

Pathology shows <u>amyloid</u>

Associated with:
MEN IIa
MEN IIb
Familial MTC only
Sporadic forms (75%; not associated with family history)

MEN IIb and **sporadic** forms have worst prognosis

Usually is the **1st manifestation** of MEN IIa and MEN IIb

From **parafollicular C cells**

Secrete **calcitonin** which causes diarrhea and flushing

C-cell hyperplasia is considered pre-malignant to MTC

Need to screen for **pheochromocytoma**

Patients who present w/ MTC as a palpable thyroid mass

20% already have distant met's to liver, lung, or bone

70% already have nodal disease

Pre-op w/u

Neck/Chest/Abd CT scan
Bone scan
LFT's

Needed for all patients w/ MTC presenting as a **mass**

Tx:
Patients who present w/ MTC as a palpable thyroid mass

Total thyroidectomy
Central neck node dissection
MRND on side of tumor

Patients w/ Family Hx and RET proto-oncogene without mass

Prophylactic total thyroidectomy (and central LN dissection) at age 2

Monitor calcitonin levels for disease recurrence

5-year survival – 50% (for patients who present w/ palpable thyroid mass)

Central LN neck dissection (removing all lymphatic tissue)

From internal jugular vein to internal jugular vein
Up to hyoid
Down to innominate vein (or as low as you can go)

Hurthle cell carcinoma

Pathology shows Ashkenazi cells

Tx: total thyroidectomy; MRND for clinically positive nodes

Anaplastic thyroid cancer

Very aggressive thyroid CA

Rapidly lethal

Hardly any patients survive

Tx: total thyroidectomy if resectable

Consider palliative thyroidectomy if refractory to chemo-XRT for compressive symptoms

Thyroid Lymphoma

MC Non-Hodgkins lymphoma

Frequently associated with Hashimoto's Thyroiditis

MC in women

LDH and beta-2 microglobulin predict worse prognosis

Tx: XRT for low stage tumors

Chemo-XRT for higher staged tumor

Recurrent laryngeal nerve injury

RLN innervates the laryngeal constrictor muscles

Enters these muscle from below

The right RLN enters the laryngeal constrictor muscles from a more lateral direction compared to the left (possibly increases the risk of injury)

Leave alone if symptoms are not that bad, most get better

If in **paramedian location**, pt's may have SOB, or may be totally asymptomatic with a normal voice

If in **abducted location**, patients will be hoarse and may need medialization (gelfoam often used) by ENT

Bilateral recurrent nerve injury can result in total airway obstruction if the cords go medial

If the cords go lateral, persistent aspiration is likely to result

In any case, patients with bilateral recurrent nerve injury most often need a permanent tracheostomy

The right recurrent laryngeal nerve is more likely to be non-recurrent compared to the left

Superior laryngeal nerve injury

Enters the cricothyroid muscle from above

Injury results in loss of pitch (would be noticed by an opera singer)

Parathyroid

Normal values

Calcium	8.5 –10.5
PTH	10 – 60 (pg/ml)
Phosphate:	2.5 – 5.0
Chloride	98 – 107
Parathyroid weight	60 – 80 gm
½ life of PTH	18 minutes

Primary Hyperparathyroidism

Autonomously elevated PTH
Elevated serum Ca
Elevated urine Ca (70%; normal in 30%)

Familial Hypercalcemic Hypocalciuria (defective PTH receptor)

Normal PTH (or slightly elevated)
Elevated serum Ca (only to 11 or so)
Low urine Ca (this is the key finding)

<u>NO</u> parathyroidectomy in these patients

Secondary hyperparathyroidism

Elevated PTH
Normal serum Ca
Elevated urine Ca

It is unusual to have to operate on patients with renal associated secondary hyperparathyroidism.

The most common indication is bone pain.

Breast

Benign Breast DZ

Infectious mastitis

Usually associated with breast feeding
Most common organism - Staph aureus
Tx: stop breast feeding, abx's

> If infection does not clear - Mammogram, skin/breast biopsy (need to rule out inflammatory CA of the breast)

In non-lactating women can be due to:

> Chronic inflammatory disease (actinomyces, TB, syphilis)
> Autoimmune disease (SLE)
> Cancer

In non-lactating women you need to get:

> Incisional biopsy of the skin and underlying breast tissue (along with a mammogram) to R/O cancer

Gynecomastia

> Can occur in adolescent pubertal boys (normal development) which usually recedes

Adult males

> RF's – Obesity, gonadal or germ cell tumors (produce estrogen), liver disease (failure to breakdown estrogen), reduced testosterone states (older age), marijuana, steroids, medications (cimetidine, spironolactone)

> Need to work up the above possibilities (i.e. LFT's, testicular exam, review medications)

> Should be bilateral o/w need to suspect CA and get a mammogram and a BX

Breast Cancer

Stage I – T1, N0, M0

Stage IIa – T0-1, N1, M0 or T2, N0, M0

Stage IIb – T2, N1, M0 or T3, N0, M0

Stage IIIa – T0-3, N2, M0 or T3, N1, M0

Stage IIIb – any T4 or N3 tumors

Stage IV – M1

5-YS:
Stage I – 90%
Stage II – 75%
Stage III – 50%
Stage IV – 15%

Nodes

Level I – lateral to pectoralis minor
Level II – beneath pectoralis minor
Level III – medial to pectoralis minor
Rotter's nodes – between pectoralis major and minor

Only need to sample level I (and some say level II) nodes

Nodes are most important prognostic staging factor (others include tumor size, grade, PR and ER status)

Larger tumors more like to have positive nodes

0 nodes positive	80% 5-YS
4+ nodes positive	40% 5-YS

You are not trying to remove all the cancer with axillary lymph node dissection for breast cancer, you are trying to stage the patient

With melanoma, you are trying to remove all of the melanoma (you take level III nodes with an axillary lymph node dissection for melanoma)

Treatment of the breast cancer primary:

Lumpectomy/XRT with sentinel lymph node biopsy or axillary lymph node dissection or;

Modified radical mastectomy

If patient has metastatic disease, no resection (just chemo-XRT and Tamoxifen) unless to palliate (i.e. inflammatory breast CA)

Chemotherapy for breast cancer (is given before XRT)

CMF - Cyclophosphamide (s/e's - hemorrhagic cystitis), methotrexate, and 5FU or;

AC - Adriamycin (s/e's - cardiomyopathy) and cyclophosphamide
Max dose of Adriamycin – 500 mg/cm^2 body surface area

4 cycles, 28 days each usual

Positive nodes

> **ER or PR positive** – chemo and Tamoxifen
> **ER and PR negative** – chemo

Negative nodes

> **>1 cm**

>> **ER or PR positive** – chemo and Tamoxifen
>> **ER and negative** – chemo

> **<1 cm and negative nodes** – Tamoxifen if ER positive

XRT for breast cancer

6 weeks, 10 minutes/d
5000 rads total
Just **decreases local recurrence**; no survival benefit

Chemo-tx is thought to act as an XRT sensitizer

81

Breast CA with Pregnancy*

1st trimester options:

MRM (best option)
Therapeutic abortion and lump/ALND (or SLNBx), XRT

Tumor < 1 cm → perform lumpectomy w/ ALND (if nodes negative, you're done)

2nd trimester options:

MRM (best option)
Therapeutic abortion and lump/ALND (or SLNBx), XRT

If after 20 weeks:
> Can perform **lumpectomy, ALND** (<u>NO</u> SLNB) and give **chemo** for 12 weeks while pregnant
> Have to accept 2%/trimester incidence of teratogenic effects for 2nd and 3rd trimesters
> Wait 6 weeks after chemo
> Deliver child
> Then XRT after delivery

Tumor < 1 cm → perform lumpectomy w/ ALND (if nodes negative, you're done)

3rd trimester options:

MRM (best option)
Therapeutic abortion and lump/ALND (or SLNBx), XRT

Can perform **lumpectomy, ALND** (<u>NO</u> SLNBx) and start **chemo**
> Have to accept 2% incidence of teratogenic effect in 3rd trimester
> Deliver child
> Then XRT after delivery

If < 6 weeks until delivery → can perform **lumpectomy** w/ **ALND** (<u>NO SLNBx</u>); give postpartum chemo and XRT

Tumor < 1 cm → perform lumpectomy w/ ALND (if nodes negative, you're done)

No XRT while pregnant (this is the main issue dictating the pathway above)

Chemotx –risk of malformation in $1^{st}/2^{nd}/3^{rd}$ trimesters is 40%/2%/2%

Need discussion w/ pt on **case by case** basis

No breastfeeding after delivery w/ CA

*These are the contemporary therapeutic strategies for this problem. A physician may not agree with these strategies but nonetheless they are the current strategies.

Male Breast Cancer

<1% of all breast CA

Almost always **ductal**

Poorer prognosis because of late presentation

Have ↑ed pectoral muscle involvement

R/O gynecomatia (bilateral)

RF's - steroids, XRT, family history, Klinefelter's Syndrome

90% of these tumors have estrogen receptors

Tx: MRM and Tamoxifen
   Post-op chemo for appropriate lesions (size > 1 cm or positive nodes)

Inflammatory breast CA (T4 disease)

Very aggressive → median survival of 36 months

Skin changes (peau d' orange), fungating mass, pain

Tx: Incisional breast Bx – will show inflammatory breast CA

Need full pre-op w/u for metastatic DZ

Although would likely still do mastectomy for comfort measures

Chest/abdominal/pelvic CT and **LFT's**

Consider bone scan and brain MRI

1st give **chemotherapy** (4 cycles; could also give XRT at this stage)

2nd **MRM** (send **skin margins for frozen section**, may need to raise skin flaps)

3rd **chemotherapy again** (4 cycles) and **XRT** (no XRT if you have already had maximum dose pre-op)

Chest wall attachment w/ breast CA (T4 disease)

Need full pre-op w/u for metastatic DZ

Chest/abdominal/pelvic CT and **LFT's**

Consider bone scan and brain MRI

No metastatic disease →

1st **give chemotherapy** (4 cycles)

2nd **MRM** and **chest wall resection**

Will need thoracotomy for this
Outline area of resection on chest wall
Try to remove the lesion en bloc (rib cutters)
Can remove associated lung if necessary
If > 5 cm (3 or more ribs) of chest wall taken, you will
    need to place a marlex (or methymethacralate) mesh
    to reconstruct chest wall

3rd **chemotherapy again** (4 cycles) and **XRT**

Metastatic disease → just go w/ **chemo-XRT**

Supra-clavicular nodes or internal mammary nodal involvement (N3 disease)

Need full pre-op w/u for metastatic DZ

Chest/abdominal/pelvic CT and **LFT's**

Consider bone scan and brain MRI

If disease limited to N3 nodes

1st **Give chemotherapy** (4 cycles)

2nd See how pt responds to chemotherapy by re-staging them w/ **chest/abdominal/pelvic CT** and **LFT's**:

If pt has a good response → MRM, then chemotherapy again (4 cycles) and XRT

If pt does not have a good response → just chemotherapy again (4 cycles) and XRT

If metastatic disease → just go w/ **chemo-XRT**

Lumpectomy and XRT for CA- need 1 cm margin

Absolute Contraindications

2 or more primaries in separate quadrants
Positive margins despite re-resection (can re-resect for negative margins)
Pregnancy
Previous XRT that would result in excessive total XRT dose

Relative contraindications

Unacceptable cosmetic result from large tumor
Scleroderma or **SLE**
Diffuse calcifications that are malignant appearing (need mastectomy)

Results of lumpectomy with XRT

2-3% chance of **local recurrence** (some say 10%)
Usually occurs within 2 years of 1st operation
Need salvage MRM for local recurrence
No real difference in **survival** compared to MRM
Can be done under local
Need good F/U

XRT for breast cancer

Complications of XRT

Erythema and local skin changes (ulceration)
Rib fractures
Radiation pneumonitis
Soft tissue sarcoma
Breast CA (ipsilateral or contra-lateral)

Contraindications to XRT

Scleroderma (can cause skin fibrosis and necrosis)
Previous XRT to that area that would result in excessive dose
Lupus (a relative contraindication)
Active rheumatoid arthritis (a relative contraindication)

XRT after mastectomy indications

Primary with skin or chest wall involvement
Primary tumor had positive margins
Tumors that are >5 cm (T3)
Inflammatory CA if not done pre-op
Advanced nodal disease
    Extracapsular invasion
    Fixed axillary nodes (N2)
    Internal mammary nodes (N3)
    > 4 nodes positive
Inflammatory CA (if not given pre-op)

Local recurrence after lumpectomy

Need to rule out metastatic disease in these patients (re-stage them aggressively)

Need salvage MRM for local recurrence (chemo-XRT alone if they have local recurrence with metastatic disease)

Important to remember you need negative margins following lumpectomy before starting XRT to help prevent recurrences.

BRCA gene + family history = 60% lifetime risk of breast CA
(autosomal dominant)

BRCA I
Ovarian CA – 40% lifetime risk
Male Breast CA – 1% lifetime risk

BRCA II
Ovarian CA – 10% lifetime risk
Male Breast CA – 10% lifetime risk

50% will get CA in the other breast w/ CA in the 1st breast

TAH and BSO w/ BRCA gene → ↓'s risk of breast CA 70%

Bilateral prophylactic mastectomy w/ BRCA gene →↓'s risk of breast CA 90%

Bilateral prophylactic mastectomy and **TAH and BSO** w/ BRCA gene→
↓'s risk of breast CA 95%

Screening mammograms starting at age 35

Yearly pelvic exam and **pelvic U/S** starting at age 25

Considerations for prophylactic mastectomy

1. Family history + BRCA gene

2. LCIS

Also need one of following:

High patient anxiety

Poor patient access for follow-up

Difficult lesion to follow

Patient preference

Tamoxifen

1% risk of blood clots

0.1% risk of endometrial CA

Dose is 20 mg/d for 5 years

Need to have positive ER or PR receptors to have benefit

Reduces annual odds of breast cancer recurrence by approximately 50%

Reduces the annual odds of death from breast cancer by approximately 25%

Thoracic

Lung CA

Most important prognostic indicator (w/o metastases) – nodes

Most common site of metastasis - brain

5-year survival without resection 10%

5-year survival with resection 30%

MC lung cancer - adenocarcinoma (<u>not</u> squamous)

T3 tumors are considered resectable (chest wall, diaphragm, pericardium) although you may need reconstruction

N2 tumors are not considered resectable – these patients should receive chemo-XRT (although in some protocols, patients who had a good response to chemo-XRT may then be considered for resection)

Evaluation for lung surgery:

Need predicted postoperative **FEV₁** that is **> 0.8** (or at least 40% of predicted value)

Forced expiratory volume in 1 sec

If it's close → get quantitative V/Q scan to see contribution of that portion of lung to overall pulmonary perfusion

It is based on the perfusion portion of the V/Q scan; if low perfusion on the side you are contemplating resecting, you may still be able to resect

Need predicted postoperative **DLCO >11–12** ml/min/mmHg CO (at least 50% of predicted value)

Represents carbon monoxide diffusion capacity

Value based on pulmonary capillary surface area, Hgb content, and alveolar architecture

No resection if pre-op **pCO2 > 45** or **pO2 < 60** at rest or if the patient is on **home O2**

No resection if pre-op **VO2 max < 10ml/min/kg** (exercise oxygen consumption)

Chest wall resection

Define your boundaries on the outside of the chest

Rib cutters; disarticulate the ribs from the spine

Posterior defects up to 10 cm require no special closure (scapula covers it)

Anterior defects up to 5 cm require no special closure

If defect too large, need marlex, Gortex, or methylmethacralate to reconstruct the chest wall

Pancoast tumor

Tumor invades apex of chest wall

Patients have either:

Horner's syndrome (invasion of sympathetic chain→ptosis, miosis, anhydrosis) and/or;

Ulnar nerve symptoms (invasion of brachial plexus)

Although considered T4 disease, is <u>not</u> an absolute contra-indication to surgery

If it is just invasion of the sympathetic chain or only T1/C8 of the brachial plexus, most would resect these

If the lesion is more extensive, just chemo-XRT

Bronchopleural fistula

Mortality up to 50%

Risk factors:

> Wider resection (pneumonectomy vs. lobectomy)
> CA in stump
> Pre-op XRT
> DM
> Mediastinal lymphadenectomy (devascularization)

50% occur after pneumonectomy

75% on right

Sx

> Serosanguinous sputum (early)
>
> Infected sputum production (late)
>
> Blood tinged sputum
>
> Falling air-fluid level in post-pneumonectomy lung space w/ new contralateral infiltrate virtually diagnostic

Tx

> Place chest tube and perform bronchoscopy to confirm dx
>
> Affected side down to avoid contaminating contra-lateral lung

< 1 week after surgery

> Likely secondary to technical problem
>
> Tx: reop; buttress stump w/ intercostal muscle flap

> 10 days after surgery

> Likely associated w/ infection (empyema that eroded into bronchus)
>
> Initially place chest tube and start Abx's

If previous lobectomy, CT likely all that will be required if found soon enough

If previous pneumonectomy, requires more extensive procedure (washout and buttress stump w/ intercostal flap)

Atelectasis

MC complication following lobectomy

Tx: incentive spirometry; have the patient walk

Bronchoscopy to look for and clear mucus plugging

If already on the ventilator, may need to ↑ TV's

Massive hemoptysis (> 600 cc/24 hrs)

Causes - fungus ball, abscess, bronchiectasis (CF), tumor, AVF

Bleeding usually from high pressure **bronchial arteries**

Initial Tx:

Turn pt to bleeding side down, no sedation

Go to OR for rigid bronch

Find the side that is bleeding (find which **lobe** if possible)

Most important aspect is to protect contralateral lung (pt's die of asphixyation, not hemorrhage)

Can use **Epi injection, cautery,** and **thrombin** to try and stop the bleeding

Fogarty balloon the bleeding side and **mainstem intubate** the good side if not controllable → can leave this Fogarty in indefinitely

Can also place a **dual lumen tube**

T and C for 6 units, correct coags

If you can resect the lesion → **thoracotomy**

If rsxn not really an option due to insufficient pulm reserve (i.e. cystic fibrosis pts) → **angio**

Pt's die of asphyxiation

Thoracic outlet syndrome

Neurologic involvement most common symptom

Most common anatomic abnormality – cervical rib

Most common cause of symptoms – brachial plexus irritation

Empyema– has 3 stages

Exudative

Swelling of pleura w/ low viscosity and cellular count

Tx: **chest tube** (send drainage for **culture and cytology**), **Abx's**

Fibrinopurulent (transitional phase)

Heavy fibrin deposits w/ turbid or purulent fluid; PMN's ↑

Tx: **chest tube** (send drainage for **cultures and cytology**), **Abx's**

Organizing (chronic phase)

In-growth of fibroblasts and capillaries w/ lung trapping by collagen

Lung no longer able to be expanded → Thick pus, thick fibrous peel

Occurs in 3-4 week period

Tx: **decortication** (visceral and parietal peel removed) ± muscle flap

Send fluid for **cultures and cytology**

Abx's, nutrition

If can't tolerate decortication, can place Eloesser flap

In general, decortication seldom required →most pts w/ parapneumonic empyema tx'd before process reaches chronic organizing phase (should be reserved for pts w/ obvious tx failures)

Pts w/ significant underlying lung DZ may also need **lung resection**

TPA therapy has been increasingly used for empyema

Lung Abscess

Necrotic area

Most commonly associated w/ aspiration (alcoholics)

Most commonly in superior segment of RLL and posterior segment of RUL

Chest CT can help differentiate empyema from lung abscess

Tx: Abx's alone are 95% successful

CT guided drainage if that fails

Surgery if above fails or cannot rule out cancer (> 6 cm, failure to resolve after 6 weeks)

Chylothorax post-op

Fluid milky white

Contains ↑**lymphocytes and TAG's** (> 110 mL/ul)

Sudan red stains fat

Tx: 3-4 weeks of conservative therapy → **chest tube, NPO** and **TPN**

If that fails, surgery w/ ligation of thoracic duct on right side low in mediastinum (80% successful) if secondary to trauma or iatrogenic injury (located between esophagus and vertebral bodies)

For **malignant causes of chylothorax** (lymphoma MC), can perform mechanical or talc pleurodesis (less successful than above)

Paraneoplastic syndromes

Squamous cell carcinoma of the lung – PTH-related peptide

Small cell carcinoma of the lung – ACTH, ADH

Most common paraneoplastic syndrome

Vascular

Popliteal artery aneurysms

Most common peripheral aneurysm

Patients have prominent popliteal pulses

Can be caused by atherosclerosis or congenital degeneration of arterial wall media

50% **bilateral**

50% have associated **aneurysm elsewhere** (AAA, femoral)

Most commonly get **thrombosis (MC)** or **emboli** w/ limb ischemia; not really prone to rupture

Leg pain can be from compression or ischemia

Surgery for all popliteal aneurysms (> 2 cm aneurysmal)

U/S is diagnostic study of choice

Tx: exclude aneurysm and bypass

Splenic artery aneurysms

Most common visceral aneurysm

More common in women, 1-2% risk of rupture

Repair if **symptomatic,** if patient is **pregnant,** or if found in **women of childbearing age**

High rate of pregnancy-related rupture – usually **3rd trimester**

Diameter >2 cm considered aneurysmal

Tx: can just be excluded (good collaterals)

RF's: fibrodysplasia, portal HTN, inflammatory DZ (ipancreatitis)

105

Thrombolytic therapy

Best indication is for thrombi < 2 weeks old

Thrombi older than that are more likely to be organized

It is easier to lyse clots in prosthetic grafts compared to vein bypasses because organization of the thrombus is slower in prosthetic grafts

Can use TPA, streptokinase, urokinase

Need to follow fibrinogen levels

If less than 100, should hold the thrombolytics

AV fistula for hemodialysis

Early failure due to technical problems (most commonly)

Dx: Get a fistulogram to help figure out problem

Fix venous problem w/ a PTFE patch hood over the anastomosis or use an interposition graft and go distal to the site of stenosis

Late failure

Is most commonly due to **intimal hyperplasia** on the venous side of the graft

Arm swelling after AVF

Results from venous HTN

Initial Tx: elevation of arm, as collaterals develop the swelling goes down

Persistence of major swelling suggests obstruction of a major outflow vein (axillary, subclavian, innominate)

Need angiogram of shunt run-off

Tx options:

Extend fistula to unobstructed vein
PTA of stenotic area
New site (last resort)

Infection - early (MC from contamination at time of surgery)

Superficial – local wound care and abx's

Deep – graft removal

Infection – late (MC from needle puncture from HD)

Can often salvage the graft or at least part of the graft by excision of infected part and bypass through non-infected area

Pseudoaneurysm in AVF graft

Usually forms from a needle stick

Tx: **open site and place stitch in hole**

If extensive may need interposition graft

Seroma following AVF graft placement

MC along arterial side

Tx:
>Percutaneous drainage
>Thrombin injection
>Consider pseudocapsule rsxn or new tunnel if persistent

Extremity ischemia following AVF graft placement

Mild form

Sx's – cold, numbness, pain in hand w/ HD

Usually reverses in a few weeks after starting HD

Severe form

Sx's can start immediately after placing graft

Usually associated w/ upper arm graft

Can be associated w/ arterial obstruction proximal to graft

Tx: Check for arterial obstruction proximally (angio)

Graft banding to improve flow to the extremity (to preserve graft)

Graft ligation (last resort)

Pseudoaneurysms

Can form after placing bypass grafts

Most commonly related to technical error (not getting full
thickness bites with suture)

Can cause massive late hemorrhage following placement of bypass
graft (due to rupture)

Need to repair pseudoaneurysms related to surgery

Pseudoaneuryms that follow puncture of an artery (i.e. coronary
cath lab femoral artery puncture)

Pressure usually resolves the problem

If continues to bleed, go with U/S guided thrombin injection

Surgery with a stitch at the puncture site if the above fail

Complications following Aorto-bifemoral repair of AAA

Major vein injury w/ cross-clamp – retro-aortic renal vein

Impotence in ⅓ secondary to disruption of autonomic nerves and blood flow to the pelvis

Mortality – 5% (elective)

Most common cause of acute death – MI

Most common cause of late death - renal failure

Graft infection– 1%

Pseudoaneurysm – 1%

Most common late complication - atherosclerotic occlusion

Leg ischemia after ABF repair

Need to look for a technical problem w/ **thrombosis or embolus**

Heparin, fluid resuscitation, back to OR

Doppler to find level of obstruction after prepping

Re-open incision and **doppler** proximal and distal to anastomosis:

If nothing wrong w/ anastomosis → likely have embolic problem

Open anastomosis
Fogarty back and forth; **heparin flushes** to remove clot
Want **2 consecutive passes** w/ good back flow

If anastomosis is the problem (thrombotic problem)

Re-do anastomosis w/ possible enlargement w/ bovine pericardium or GSV patch

Can also place a patch and go to a new site
Still need to Fogarty and heparin flush until 2 good passes

Completion angiogram in OR

Feel pulse to make sure you got it back

Feel calfs and consider **fasciotomy** for ischemia > 4 hours (clinical exam and compartment pressures for compartment syndrome)

Check urine myoglobin if worried about myonecrosis

Check K and H → watch for washout electrolyte problems and hypotension

Ischemic colitis following ABF repair

Bloody diarrhea

Inferior mesenteric artery likely ligated with repair

Blood flow to the left colon now impaired

Dx: sigmoidoscopy

Middle and lower rectum spared from ischemia

Make sure to go up to splenic flexure

Tx:
If the bowel wall is necrotic, go to OR for colectomy

If the bowel wall is not necrotic, follow exam for peritoneal signs or worsening clinical status

Aortoduodenal fistula following ABF repair

Usually > 6 months since surgery

Classically presents as **herald bleed** with hematemesis

Dx: Abd CT (fat stranding, possible contrast leak into bowel; thickend bowel wall)

MC in 3rd or 4th portion of duodenum near proximal suture line

Tx: Excise graft

Axillary femoral bypass with fem-fem cross-over or bilateral Ax-fem

Resection of graft with aortic stump closure

Repair duodenum

Chylous Ascites following ABF repair

Tx: re-op to ligate the cisterna chili area

Located to the right of the aorta near the right renal artery

Peritoneal venous shunt an alternative

Infected graft following ABF Repair

MC with grafts going to the groins

Tx: Excise graft

Axillary femoral bypass with fem-fem cross or bilateral Ax-fem

Resection of graft with aortic stump closure

Plavix – has been shown to improve graft patency following lower extremity bypass

Malperforans ulcer

Occurs at the metatarsal heads

Most commonly at the second MTP joint

Occurs most often is diabetics

Involves osteomyelitis

Tx: Non-weight bearing

Debridement of cartilage back to bone at the metatarsal head

Antibiotics

Angiogram to assess for possible revascularization

Severe leg swelling following lower extremity bypass

MC cause in 1st 24 hours post-op– edema from reperfusion injury

MC cause in late post-op period – DVT

Normal venous Doppler ultrasound

Augmentation of blood flow with distal compression or release of proximal compression

Graft Infection

Most common in grafts going below groin

Most sensitive test for diagnosis of graft infection - tagged white blood cell scan

Usually need to excise the graft and bypass through a new area (non-anatomic bypass)

Esophagus

Esophageal cancer

Spreads quickly along **submucosal lymphatic channels**

Criteria for resection:

> **Have to be able to tolerate surgery** (pulmonary, cardiac, liver, nutrition assessment)
>
> **Have resectable DZ** (<u>no</u> met's)

Symptoms: dysphagia and **weight loss**

Labs and studies:

> **Barium Swallow** – usually shows mass (best 1st test for dysphasia or odynophagia)
>
> **EGD** w/ Bx (to get Dx) and **EUS** (to assess depth)
>
> Once you make the CA Dx, assess for **resectability** and whether or not pt can **tolerate operation**
>
> **Neck, Chest, and Abdomen CT** (look at adrenal and liver)
>
> Supraclavicular or celiac adenopathy, liver mass, adrenal mass, lung mass → need to Bx
>
> > **Metastatic DZ** to any of these areas excludes resection
>
> **Bronchoscopy** for upper 2/3 tumors to make sure it is not growing into the trachea
>
> **PFT's** – poor PFT's, go w/ trans-hiatal esophagectomy

Unresectability

Hoarseness (RLN)
Horner's syndrome (unlike lung CA)
Phrenic nerve involvement
Malignant pleural effusion
Malignant fistula
Airway invasion
Vertebral invasion

Distant metastases – most go to lung or liver; <u>contraindication to esophagectomy</u>

Nodal DZ outside the area of resection (i.e. SMA, celiac nodes or supraclavicular nodes → considered M DZ) – contra-indication to esophagectomy

Malignant fistulas – most die within 3 months due to aspiration

Pre-operative XRT and chemotx

May down-stage tumors and make them resectable

Seems to increase survival for > T1 tumors (anything greater than invasion of submucosa)

Consider for tumors that are > T1 DZ

Cisplatnin and 5-FU (usually 6 cycles)

Adenocarcinoma #1 esophageal cancer – <u>not</u> squamous

Adenocarcinoma – usually in lower 1/3 of esophagus

Post-op tx

Chemotherapy – 5-FU and cisplatnin (use if lymphatics involved or full thickness lesion)

XRT – has been shown to been somewhat effective for local recurrence (better when combined with chemotherapy)

Esophageal Perforation

Most need operative repair – try to avoid esophagectomy if at all possible and just repair the perforation

Contained perforations without substantial systemic effects can be treated conservatively (Abx's, IVF's, serial CXR/AXR's, repeat gastrograffin/thin barium swallows)

Perforations associated w/ **distal obstruction** from intrinsic DZ have increased incidence of repair breakdown (i.e.achalasia)

Need to relieve the obstruction at the time of repair

Perforations associated w/ **intrinsic esophageal DZ that cannot be treated more conservatively**:

Cancer
Non-dilatable esophageal stricture
Severe caustic injury causing mediastinitis
Extensive esophageal devitalization associated w/ gunshot wounds

Tx: Need **esophagectomy** (probably the best choice) or:

Can perform **exclusion and diversion**

Cervical esophagostomy for spit fistula
Staple the esophagus at the level of the stomach
Place chest tubes

If patient is stable with minimal contamination, possible to do gastric pull-up at same time of esophagectomy

Late perforations (> 24 hours) with **extensive mediastinitis** – tx options:

Esophageal diversion and exclusion or:

Esophagectomy and hook up at a later date

Esophageal Diverticulum

Zenker's Diverticulum

From failure of the upper esophageal sphincter to relax with swallowing

Pressure pushes the mucosa out-pouching

False diverticula

Usually **posterior**

Sx: dysphagia, choking, halitosis

Dx: **barium swallow studies**

No **EGD** - risk for perforation

Tx: **cricopharyngeal myotomy** (key)

Diverticula can either be resected or suspended (so that it empties into the esophagus)

Usually a left cervical incision

Leave drains in

Gastrograffin followed by thin barium swallow the next day to check for a leak

Leiomyoma

#1 benign tumor of the esophagus

Usually present with dysphagia

These are submucosal

Barium Swallow used for diagnosis

Need endoscopy R/O cancer (do not biopsy through the mucosa –
   scarring will develop, making later enucleation difficult)

Most commonly in the lower ⅔ of esophagus

Tx: **>5 cm or symptoms** → enucleation; through thoracotomy

Esophageal Strictures

R/O malignancy
Serial dilatation
May need to replace the esophagus if non-dilatable

Stomach

Postgastrectomy complications

Dumping syndrome

Occurs after gastrectomy or vagotomy and pyloroplasty

From rapid entry of carbohydrates into the small bowel

90% of cases resolve with medically

2 parts

1. Hyperosmotic load leads to osmotic fluid shift into bowel (**hypotension and diarrhea**)

2. Insulin increases significantly and **hypoglycemia occurs** (2nd phase rarely occurs)

Tx: small meals that are high protein, low-fat, and low-carbohydrate

Avoid liquids with meals

Avoid lying down after meals

Octreotide before meals is effective in many

Surgical options (rarely necessary)

Roux-en-Y gastrojejunostomy (convert BI or BII to this)

Can increase the size of the stomach pouch with jejunum

Can also reverse a piece of jejunum so that the transit time is slower

Duodenal stump blowout

Lateral duodenostomy tube (just stick this in the hole and sew purse-string around it)

Gastro-jejunostomy and pyloric exclusion to allow the area to heal

Drains

Feeding J-tube

Motilin receptor

Erythromycin acts as a pro-kinetic by binding to this receptor

Motilin receptor is located in the **stomach** (MC area - antrum), duodenum, and colon

H. pylori

CLO test detects urease released from H-pylori

Biopsy on EGD needs to be from the **antrum**

Liver

Hepatocellular CA (Hepatic sarcoma, Cholangiosarcoma – similar tx)

Risk factors – hepatitis, ETOH, primary sclerosing cholangitis

5-YS – 30% (with resection)

Tumors are often unresectable secondary to:

Cirrhosis
Portahepatic involvement
Metastases

Usually need **formal rsxn** and a **1-cm margin**

HCC w/u

Chest/Abdomen/Pelvic CT scan (vessel involvement, portal nodes, or met's)

Does pt have **cirrhosis** (if significant, contra-indication to rsxn)

Diagnostic laparoscopy before laparotomy

Hepatic cystadenoma/-carcinoma (rare)

U/S will show **papillary-like fronds** within the cyst itself

Can be **complex** (more likely malignant)

Mucin production

Tx: formal resection unless cystadenoma (wedge)

Biliary cystadenoma/-carcinoma (rare)

U/S will show characteristic **very thick cyst wall**

Biliary cystadenoma

Fine calcifications, septated

pre-malignant, slow-growing

MC in women

Biliary Cystadenocarcinoma

As above but invasive w/ course calcifications

Tx: formal resection unless cystadenoma (wedge)

<u>Liver resection</u>

Part of the difficulty in assessing whether or not liver tumors are resectable is deciding on whether or not you are going to leave enough liver for the patient to survive

One of the best prognostic tests for determining quantitatively the amount of liver reserve in patients being evaluated for resection is MEGX test

MEGX test

Inject Lidocaine into the patient

Measure the production of monoethylglycinexylidid (MEGX)

Low production of this metabolite indicates poor liver reserve

Biliary System

Cholecystitis

ERCP Indications (suspected common bile duct stone):

Jaundiced patient

Cholangitis (RUQ pain, fever, jaundice)

Gallstone pancreatitis

Elevated bilirubin (can also be due to primary liver DZ)

Significantly elevated AST or ALT (can also be due to primary liver DZ)

Stone in CBD on ultrasound

Large stones in CBD on intra-op cholangiogram

Need to remove these

Small stone in CBD on intra-op cholangiogram

Leave alone

Small stones will almost always pass

Also have the option of post-op ERCP if it does become obstructive (ERCP 98% effective at removing stones)

Retained CBD stone after placement of T-tube

Can use stone retrieval device through T-tube

ERCP

Treatment of choice for late presenting common bile duct stones

Involves:

Sphincterotomy

Tools and baskets can then be used to remove the stone

Risk's:

Bleeding from CBD or duodenum

Severe pancreatitis

Perforation of the bile duct or duodenum

Emphysematous gallbladder

Gas producing organisms in the gallbladder wall

Diabetics are at increased risk

Caused by *Clostridium perfringens* usually

Sx: Rapidly progressing, severe, abdominal pain

Nausea and vomiting

Sepsis

Tx: cholecystectomy on an emergent basis

Broad spectrum antibiotics at 1st (although **high dose PCN** is the classic treatment for clostridium infection)

Bile duct injuries intra-op during cholecystectomy

1st sign is often **bile staining** at time of cholecystectomy

Make sure **cystic duct clip** has not fallen off

Look for location of the bile drainage

Get an **IOC (intra-op cholangiogram) to help find the leak**

Intraoperative CBD injury

> < 50% circumference of CBD or hepatic duct, perform primary repair

> All other cases (which is the majority of injuries) hepatico-jejunostomy or choledocho-jejunostomy

Duct of Luschka

> < 2 mm duct that is a direct connection of the liver to the GB

> These can leak bile at the end of the case

> Tx: ligate the duct

Accessory right posterior hepatic duct

> From segments 6 and/or 7

> Enters the CBD separately (need to look for these in the triangle of Calot)

> **If < 2 mm**

>> Just ligate

May need **IOC** to look for attachment to CBD (would need to ligate that as well)

If > 2 mm

Will need hepatico-jejunostomy (attach the anomalous duct to a jejunal loop)

Need **IOC** to look for attachment to CBD (would need to ligate)

Gallbladder CA

Rare tumors although they are the most common CA of the biliary tract

Different subtypes – adenocarcinoma, clear cell, papillary, etc.

Papillary has the best prognosis

Most common site of metastasis – liver

Porcelain gallbladder

> This is a risk factor for gallbladder CA (15%)
>
> Patient with a porcelain gallbladder should undergo cholecystectomy

Spreads to **segments IV and V initially**

1st nodes to be involved are the cystic duct nodes (right side)

Tx: **CA limited to the mucosa (stage I)**

> Cholecystectomy only

CA into the muscle (stage II)

> Wide resection at segments IV and V (2–3 cm margins; some just perform segmentectomies to avoid bleeding)
>
> Regional lymphadenectomy (need to include portal triad)

High incidence of **tumor implants** at trocar sites

Laparoscopic approach contraindicated

5-year survival – 5%

Pancreas

Secretin

Increases bile flow

Increases pancreatic HCO3- release

Inhibition of HCL and gastrin release

Notably, gastrin will go up with secretin injection in patients with gastrinoma

Acts on pancreatic ductal cells

CCK

Causes gallbladder contraction

Pancreatic enzyme release

Relaxation of the sphincter of Oddi

Some increase in intestinal motility

Acts primarily on pancreatic acinar cells

CCK and secretin

Majority is released from cells located in the duodenum

Pancreatic pseudocysts

Usually in patients with **chronic pancreatitis**

Pain most common symptom

> Can also get fever, weight loss, bowel obstruction from compression

Non-epithelialized cyst

Usually in head of pancreas

Expectant management up to 3 months

> Need to allow the pseudocyst to mature

> May need TPN if unable to eat

Only need to treat for **continued symptoms or if growing**

Tx: Symptomatic or growing pseudocyst after 3 months - need MRCP or ERCP to check for duct involvement.

> Duct involved - will need **cystogastrostomy (endoscopic or open)**

> Duct not involved – can try just percutaneous drainage of pseudocyst 1st (occasionally works); if that fails will need cysto-gastrostomy

Percutaneous or open cysto-gastrostomy for pancreatic pseudocyst

Need to make sure this is not CA 1st

Take Bx of wall at time of cysto-gastrostomy

If patient does not have a history of chronic pancreatitis – very suspicious for CA

Complications from a pancreatic pseudocyst

Small bowel obstruction from compression

Infection

Portal vein or splenic vein thrombosis

Major bleeding

Severe bleeding from either a pancreatic pseudocyst, debrided pancreas from infected necrosis, or after whipple

Go to angio before OR and try to embolize

Operating on patients in the above scenarios is extremely difficult so you want to avoid it

Pancreatic fistulas

Majority close spontaneously (especially if low output < 200 cc/d)

Try to wait it out

Dx: send fluid for **amylase and lipase**

Tx: control drainage (ostomy)

> **Abx's** (zosyn 3.35 IV Q 6) for 1st week (
>
> **NPO**
>
> **TPN or distal feedings**
>
> **Octreotide** (to decrease pancreatic output)
>
> **Follow electrolytes**
>
> **Abd CT to R/O abscess or fluid collection**
>
> **Send fluid for culture and cytology** (is this a CA recurrence?)

If failure to resolve w/ medical management after 6-8 weeks →**ERCP, sphincterotomy, temporary stent** to try and get it to close

If that fails after 6-8 weeks, for distal lesions perform **distal pancreatectomy**

Possibly **whipple** for proximal lesions

Do <u>not</u> rush to operate on these patients

Splenic vein thrombosis

Chronic pancreatitis most common cause of splenic vein thrombosis

Can get bleeding from gastric varices that form as collaterals (do not form esophageal collaterals)

Tx: splenectomy (for bleeding gastric varices not associated with esophageal varices)

Acute pancreatitis

Stones and **ETOH** most common causes

Mortality rate 10%

Hemorrhagic pancreatitis mortality rate - 50%

Pancreatitis without obvious cause (no stones or ETOH)

Need to worry about **malignancy**

Hyponatremia associated w/ pancreatitis

From hyperlipidemia (pseudo-hyponatremia)

Necrosis (and infected necrosis)

Generally leave sterile necrosis alone

Get CT guided sample if fluid is suspicious (tiny air bubbles) to see if its infected → if you think its infected, proceed w/ OR and scooping out dead pancreas, leave drains

CT guided drainage of infected necrosis of the pancrease is not effective

Usually GNR's

May need multiple debridements

Insulinoma

HPI: Whipple's triad

1) **Fasting hypoglycemia** (< 50)

2) **Sx's of hypoglycemia**, (palpitations, ↑ed HR, and diaphoresis)

3) **Relief with glucose**

Dx: Insulin to glucose ratio >0 .4 after fasting

Fasting glucose **< 60**

Fasting insulin **> 24**

The above r/o liver DZ as a cause

↑ **C peptide** and **pro-insulin** → if not elevated suspect Munchausen's syndrome

Localization:

Abd CT (or MRI)

Look for liver tumors or mesothelioma on upper cuts

Octreotide scan – if having trouble localizing

Tx: Enucleate if <2 cm

Can have multiple lesions (enucleate each if < 2 cm)

Formal rsxn if >2 cm (whipple or distal pancreatectomy)

Look around for node DZ

Check serum glucose level after removal
To make sure you got the insulinoma
The 1/2 life of insulin is **4 minutes**

Gastrinoma (Zollinger-Ellison syndrome)

50% malignant
50% multiple

Gastrinoma triangle

1. Common bile duct

2. Neck of pancreas

3. Third portion of the duodenum

HPI: Refractory ulcer disease (abdominal pain)

Diarrhea (improved with H2 blockers)

Labs and studies

Always need serum gastrin level and stomach basal acid output to make Dx

Serum gastrin

Usually >200 (although not diagnostic)

> 1000's is diagnostic

Basal Acid Output

> 15 mEq/hr (no previous vagotomy) → c/w gastrinoma

> 5 mEq/hr (previous vagotomy) → c/w gastrinoma

Secretin stimulation test

Patients w/ gastrinoma will have an increase in gastrin (> 200 increase)

Normal patients have ↓ gastrin

Abd CT (or MRI) to localize; look for multiple tumors

Octreotide scan – if having trouble localizing

> May be good to get in all patients as 50% have multiple tumors; all the tumors may <u>not</u> show up on Abd CT

Tx: enucleation if <2 cm

Formal resection if >2 cm

Malignant disease → excise suspicious nodes

Can't find tumor →

> Perform duodenostomy and look inside duodenum for tumor (15% of microgastrinomas there)

Duodenal tumor – resection with primary closure

> May need Whipple if extensive

> Be sure to **check pancreas** for another primary (50% multiple)

Spleen

Postsplenectomy sepsis syndrome

Streptococcus pneumoniae (#1), haemophilus influenza, neisseria meningitides

Secondary to lack of immunity to capsulated bacteria

Highest risk - splenectomy for **hemolytic disorders or malignancy**

Vaccines needed - pneumococcus, meningococcus, H. Influenza

Give before splenectomy if possible

Splenic abscess

Mortality rate 30%

MC from remote source – endocarditis or IVDA

MC have enteric organisms in the abscess

Best tx is removal of spleen

Adrenal

Hyperaldosteronism (Conn's syndrome)

Sx's - HTN, polydipsia and polyuria

Dx for primary hyperaldosteronism:

Aldosterone:renin ratio > 400

Low serum K (usually < 3), high serum Na

High urine K

Metabolic alkalosis

Localizing studies (figuring out adenoma vs. hyperplasia):

Abd CT or MRI

NP-59 scintography - shows hyperfunctioning adrenal tissue

Helps differentiate hyperplasia from adenoma

Selective adrenal venous sampling

Captopril test and measure aldosterone →

If aldosterone level decreases after captopril → hyperplasia

If aldosterone stay the same after captopril → adenoma

Tx:

Adenoma resection has good results with adrenalectomy

Diffuse hyperplasia

Try medical therapy first using **spironolactone, calcium channel blockers** (try many types of anti-hypertensive agents), and **potassium.**

143

If bilateral resection performed (which is usually done for refractory **hypokalemia**), will need **fludrocortisone** postoperatively.

Pheochromocytoma

10% rule (all of the following occur at a rate of 10%)

Malignant
Bilateral
In children
Familial
Extra-adrenal
MEN

Extra-adrenal tumors more likely malignant

Only **adrenal pheochromocytomas** produce **epinephrine** from NE (have **PNMT enzyme**)

Sx - HTN (frequently **episodic**), HA, diaphoresis, palpitations

Dx: 24 hour urine – Epi, NE, VMA, metanephrines and nor-metanephrines (best test overall)

Serum levels – Epi, NE, VMA, metanephrines and nor-metanephrines

Clonidine suppression test – tumor doses not respond, keeps catecholamines high

CT (or MRI) can help localize tumors

MIBG scan (norepinephrine analogue) scan can help locate

<u>No</u> **venography** → can cause hypertensive crisis

Not able to localize → still proceed w/ laparotomy

Preop

Alpha-blocker first

Phenoxybenzamine (start at 10 mg/d and ramp up) or prazosin (start at 1 mg and ramp up)

Avoid hypertensive crisis by starting the alpha-blocker 1st

Start at least 2 weeks before OR and increase dose until pt has slight orthostatic hypotension

Give PO volume replacement during this time

Beta-blocker if patient has tachycardia or arrhythmias while on alpha blocker

Need to be careful with beta-blocker and give after alpha blocker → can precipitate **hypertensive crisis** (un-apposed alpha stimulation) or **heart failure** in patients with cardiomyopathy

Tx: **Have nipride, esmolol, dopamine, and phenylephrine** ready to go at the time of surgery

Have a **swan, foley, a-line**

Transabdominal approach for these (classic teaching, so that you can look at the contra-lateral adrenal for bilateral DZ or be able to handle a malignant pheochromocytoma that is invading other structures)

Many are doing these laparoscopically and relying on pre-op imaging for diagnosing bilateral or malignant DZ

10% bilateral (would look at other adrenal if doing this transabdominal)

Transabdominal approach:

Left side → Mattox maneuver (left colon and spleen)

Right side → Cattel maneuver (right colon and duodenum), also need to take down the right triangular ligament of the liver

Ligate adrenal vein first to avoid spilling catecholamines during tumor manipulation

Debulking helps symptoms in patients w/ unresectable DZ

Other sites of pheochromocytomas:

    Vertebral bodies

    Sympathetic chain ganglia (paravertebral)

    Opposite adrenal gland

    Bladder

    Aortic bifurcation (MC ectopic location) – organ of Zuckerkandl

Hypertension during removal → esmolol, nipride

Persistent hypertension after removal

    Check for other sites of pheochromocytoma as above
    Check the contra-lateral adrenal

Hypotension after removal – volume, phenylephrine

Bronchospasm after removal – albuterol, epinephrine

Other cx's – arrhythmias, intra-cerebral hemorrhage, CHF, MI

Metyrosine

    Inhibits **tyrosine hydroxylase** causing ↓ed synthesis of catecholamines

    Can be used pre-op

Small Bowel

Appendicitis Foils

Regional ileitis – 10% go on to Crohn's disease

Gastroenteritis – nausea, vomiting, diarrhea

Mucocele

MC on the **appendix**

15% have another malignancy in the abdomen

Can be benign or malignant mucinous cystadenocarcinoma

Needs resection → right hemicolectomy if malignant

Pseudomyxoma peritonei occurs w/ rupture (tumor spreads through abdomen – eventually causes bowel obstructions from tumor implants)

Carcinoid

MC site – appendix (50% of carcinoids arise here)

Ileum and rectum next most common

Carcinoid in appendix

<2 cm and not involving base → appendectomy

≥2 cm or involving base → right hemicolectomy

Presumed appendicitis but find ruptured ovarian cyst, or thrombosed ovarian vein, or regional enteritis not involving cecum
→ **still perform appendectomy**

Complications from removal of terminal ileum

↓ **B$_{12}$ and folate uptake** can result in **megaloblastic anemia**

Cobalamin	Megaloblastic anemia
(B$_{12}$)	Glossitis
Deficiency	Peripheral neuropathy
Folate	Megaloblastic anemia
Deficiency	Glossitis
	NO peripheral neuropathy

↓ **bile salt uptake** causes osmotic **diarrhea** (bile salts) and **steatorrhea** (↓ fat uptake) in colon

↓ **bile salt uptake** can result in the formation of **gallstones**

↓ **oxalate binding to Ca** secondary to increased intraluminal fat
  → more oxalate then gets absorbed in colon
  → released in urine
  → **Ca oxalate Kidney Stones (hyperoxaluria)**

Duodenal Crohn's Disease – medical tx initially

If **obstructing**, just bypass with gastro-jejunostomy (no whipple)

Intussusception in adults – MC from cecal adenocarcinoma

SB lymphoma (MC in ileum)

Tx: rsxn, chemo, XRT

Just chemo-XRT if in the duodenum

GI tract is the MC extra-nodal site for Non-Hodgkins Lymphoma (NHL)

MC – B cell

Stomach Lymphoma

Tx: chemo-XRT standard, resection possibly for just stage I only

Pancreatic Lymphoma

Tx: chemo-XRT standard

Colorectal

Colon Cancer

T1: into the submucosa

T2: into the muscularis propria

T3: into sub-serosa or non-peritonealized fat if no serosa present, or completely through the muscularis propria

T4: completely through serosa or into adjacent organs/structures or perforates the visceral peritoneum

N0: nodes negative

N1: 1–3 nodes positive

N2: ≥4 nodes positive

M1: distant metastases

Stage I	T1–2,N0,M0
Stage II	T3–4, N0, M0
Stage III	Any N1 disease
Stage IV	Any M1 disease

5-YS for colon cancer

Stage I – 95%
Stage II – 70%
Stage III – 40%
Stage IV – 5%

Chemotherapy

Stage III and IV colon CA (nodes positive or distant metastases)

→ resection, post-op chemo (or just chemo if not resecting the primary for stage IV disease) no XRT

Stage II and III rectal CA

→ pre-op or post-op chemo-XRT and resection

Stage IV rectal CA

→ chemo and XRT +/– surgery (possibly just colostomy)

Chemotherapy for all of above → 5FU and Leucovorin (6 cycles)

XRT (5000 rads)

↓'s local recurrence and improves survival when combined with chemotherapy

XRT damage – rectum most common site of injury → vasculitis, thrombosis, ulcers, strictures

Pre-op XRT and chemotherapy downstage (can have complete response) allowing LAR vs. APR

Really high risk pts → possibly chemo-XRT only tx

Follow-up

CEA (1/2 life 18 days) persistently elevated after colectomy but can't find source despite extensive w/u – 2nd look laparotomy

History and physical exam, CEA, stool guaiac, LFTs, abdominal CT, CXR – every 6 months for 3 years, then annually – 20% have recurrence

Colonoscopy yearly (mainly to check for new colon CA's; metachronous)

Liver met discovered at the time of colon resection

If really easy to remove, just wedge it out

If not really easy to remove, just take a wedge Bx and send it to path:

Finish the operation you were there to do

Re-stage the patient after 6-8 weeks (Abd and Pelvic CT, CXR, CEA, and LFT's)

If no other metastatic DZ is detected, resect the colon met

Metastases usually do <u>not</u> create more metastases

Low rectal T1 (limited to submucosa) – assess w/ **TRUS**

Can be excised trans-anally if:

<4 cm in size

Not circumferential

Negative margins (need 1 cm)

Well differentiated

No neurologic/vascular/lymphatic invasion

< 8 cm away

Otherwise patient needs APR or LAR

Place pt in Jack-Knife position; Fergusson-Hill retractor

Wound drainage post-op

Differential Diagnosis:

> **Dehiscence (or evisceration)**
> **Necrotizing fascitis**
> **Bowel leak** (< 7 days)
> **Bowel fistula** (≥ 7 days)
> **Wound infection**
> **Seroma**
> **Urine leak**

Pull out a few staples or look into the opening to **assess the fascia:**

> Have **sutures pulled through** the fascia → **if yes, you have a dehiscence** → laparotomy
>
> Does the fascia look **infected?** → **possible fascitis** → laparotomy
>
> What **type of fluid** is draining from the wound?

> 1) **Clear pink or salmon colored** – likely a **dehiscence**
>
>> Check to see if the **sutures have pulled through** and for **infection** → **if yes, OR**
>
> 2) **Yellow Pus** → likely a **wound infection**
>
>> Check to see if the **sutures have pulled through** and for **fascitis** → **if yes, OR.** If sutures are intact treat like a wound infection
>
> 3) **Gray and foul smelling** → likely **necrotizing fascitis**
>
>> Go to OR for debridement
>
> 4) **Green** → injury or leak from **small bowel**

Check to see if the **sutures have pulled through** and for **fascitis** → **if yes, OR.** If no, follow below:

< 7 days (this is a leak) → re-operate and fix the problem

≥ 7 days (this is a fistula) → conservative therapy if fascia is intact and there are no signs of fascitis (and no peritoneal signs or signs of sepsis)

5) **Brown (stool)** → injury or leak from **large bowel**

Check to see if the **sutures have pulled through** and for **fascitis** → **if yes, OR.** If no, follow below:

< 7 days (this is a leak) → re-operate

≥ 7 days (this is a fistula) → conservative therapy if fascia is intact and there are no signs of fascitis (and no peritoneal signs or signs of sepsis)

6) **Clear yellow tinged** (more likely after APR) → **urine** (send Cr to confirm)

Check to see if the **sutures have pulled through** and for **fascitis** → **if yes, OR.** If no, follow below:

< 7 days → re-operate and repair (see Trauma section for types of ureteral repair)

≥ 7 days → place drain (or ostomy) and repair in 6-8 weeks

Familial adenomatous polyposis (FAP)

Autosomal dominant

APC gene – chromosome 5

This gene is involved in cell adhesion and cytoskeletal function

Polyps do not present until puberty

Duodenal polyps → check duodenum for cancer every 2 years

Lifetime surveillance of residual rectal mucosa to check for CA

Gardner's syndrome - colon CA (APC gene) and desmoid tumors and/or osteomas

Turcot's syndrome - colon CA (APC gene) and brain tumors

Lynch syndromes (hereditary non-polyposis colon cancer)

Autosomal dominant

DNA mismatch repair gene.

Most commonly **right-sided colon cancers**

Lynch I –colon CA only

Lynch II –increased risk of ovarian, endometrial, bladder, and stomach cancer in addition to colon cancer

Amsterdam criteria

3 or more 1st degree relatives

2 generations

1 relative with cancer before age 50

Anus

Anal cancer

Association w/ **HPV** and **XRT**

Anal Canal Lesions (above dentate line)

Squamous Cell CA of Anal Canal (Type of Epidermal CA)

Sx's: pruritus, bleeding, palpable mass

Labs and Studies

Get Bx of lesion
Abd/Pelvic CT
CXR
LFT's

Tx: **chemo-XRT 1st line**

Nigro protocol

5-FU and mitomycin
XRT
Not surgery

This cures 80%.

Need to get FNA of clinically positive **inguinal nodes** and spread the XRT field to include the inguinal area if CA is present

Re-Bx the anal area in 1 month as well as inguinal FNA if patient had previous positive nodes

→ give another cycle of chemo-XRT if either is positive

Re-Bx the anal area again in 1 month as well as inguinal FNA if patient had previous positive nodes

If **anal area** still positive → APR

If **inguinal nodes** still positive → **inguinal LN dissection**

Basaloid CA, Cloacogenic CA, mucoepidermoid CA

Tx same as Squamous Cell CA

Melanoma

Hematogenous spread early; accounts for most deaths

Rectal bleeding – most common symptom

Often only lightly **pigmented or not pigmented at all**

Tx: **APR** for **thick melanoma (> 4 mm)**

Local resection for **superficial melanoma (< 1 mm)**

Intermediate melanoma (1-4 mm) – case by case basis (APR probably the safest answer)

Hemorrhoids

Tx: Fergusson-hill retractor

Resect down to the internal sphincter w/ elliptical incision in the 3 quadrants

Make sure you can insert 3 fingers after resecting hemorrhoids

Post-op fiber, stool softeners, sitz baths

MC complication – urinary retention

RF's – males, older age, increased narcotic requirement

Surgical indications – bleeding, pain, large external component

Hernias and Abdominal Wall

Sliding hernia

Visceral peritoneum coming from a retroperitoneal structure makes up part of the sac

The retroperitoneal organ is included in the herniated tissue

Ovary MC in females

Cecum MC in males

Ilioinguinal nerve injury

Most commonly injured nerve with inguinal hernia repair

Loss of cremasteric reflex

Numbness on ipsilateral scrotum and thigh

Usually injured at **external ring**

Nerve runs anterior to the cord structures

Genitofemoral nerve injury

Most commonly occurs with w/ laparoscopic hernia repair

Genital branch

Gives branches to cremaster (motor) and scrotum (sensory)

Genital branch runs posterior and inferior to the cord

Femoral branch

Goes to upper lateral thigh (sensory)
Runs lateral to iliac vessels

Femoral Hernias

Femoral canal boundaries:

Superior - inguinal ligament

Inferior – pectineal ligament

Medial – lacunar ligament (attaches to pubis; connects inguinal and pectineal ligaments)

Lateral - femoral vein

Very high risk of incarceration → may need to **divide inguinal ligament** to reduce bowel

Hernia goes under inguinal ligament

Characteristic **bulge** on anterior-medial thigh **below inguinal ligament**

Laparoscopic Ventral Hernia Repair

RF's for recurrence of ventral hernia after laparoscopic repair

Obesity
Large defects
Previous hernia repair

0.1% incidence of placing the veress needle or trocar into bowel or blood vessel

Laparoscopic Inguinal Hernia repair

Want a tension free repair

MC reason for recurrence - mesh is too small (poor tacking also common cause)

MC location for recurrence– medial portion of mesh near the pubis

Ostitis – can occur if your try to anchor the stitches to the pubic bone itself. Tx: NSAID's

Parastomal hernias

More common w/ large bowel stomas then small bowel stomas

Patients usually tolerate these well and routine repair is not recommended

Absolute indications for repair include **obstruction** and **incarceration w/ strangulation**

2 methods of repair:

stomal relocation (best choice)

prosthetic repair

facial repair (bringing the fascia together near the hernia) doesn't really work

Pseudohernia – missing the rectus and bringing the ostomy through the oblique muscle

Tx: relocate in the rectus muscle

Urology

Testicular cancer

Symptoms - painless hard mass

Labs and studies:

U/S – is it a hydrocoele? (will transluminate if so)

Chest and abdominal CT – look for met's

AFP, B-HCG, and **LDH** (correlates w/ tumor bulk)

Orchiectomy through an **inguinal incision** (<u>not</u> trans-scrotal → do not want to disrupt lymphatics)

The testicle and attached mass are the biopsy specimen

Undescended testicles (crypto-orchidism) – ↑ risk of seminoma

Seminoma

#1 testicular tumor; 10% have beta-HCG elevation

Should <u>not</u> have AFP elevation (if elevated, need to treat like non-seminomatous testicular cancer)

Spreads to retroperitoneum

Seminoma is extremely sensitive to XRT

Tx:
All stages get:

Orchiectomy
Retroperitoneal XRT (for occult retroperitoneal metastases)

Chemo (Cisplatnin, Bleomycin, Etoposide) for:

Metastatic disease
Bulky retroperitoneal disease

Surgical resection of residual metastases (after chemo-XRT)

Non-seminomatous testicular CA

AFP and **beta-HCG** – positive in 90%

Spreads to **lungs** and **retroperitoneum**

Surgical Tx

Stage I

Orchiectomy
Prophylactic **retroperitoneal node dissection** (Stage II if tumor there)

Stage II or greater:

Orchiectomy
Chemo (cisplatnin, Bleomycin, VP-16)
Surgical resection of residual metastases

Renal cell carcinoma (hypernephroma)

RF – smoking

Symptoms - Abdominal pain, abdominal mass, and hematuria (classic)

Can often diagnose renal cell carcinoma just based on CT scan characteristics (necrosis, calcifications)

1/3 have met's at time of diagnosis → wedge resection of isolated lung (MC) and colon met's

Erythrocytosis can occur secondary to ↑ erythropoietin (HTN)

Most common tumor in kidney – **metastasis from the breast**

Tx: radical nephrectomy w/ regional nodes; XRT, chemotherapy (doxorubicin based)

> **Radical nephrectomy** takes:
>
> > **Kidney**
> >
> > **Adrenal**
> >
> > **Fat**
> >
> > **Gerota's Fascia**
> >
> > **Regional nodes**
>
> Predilection for growth in the IVC, can still resect even if going up IVC → can pull the tumor thrombus out
>
> Partial nephrectomies considered only for patients who would require dialysis after nephrectomy
>
> Embolization can be used to palliate large tumors or as pre-op for large tumors to facilitate removal

Undescended testicles

Usually do not treat until 2 years old

Higher risk of testicular CA than in general population

Cancer risk stays the same even after the testicle is brought down into scrotum.

Seminoma – most common cancer associated with undescended testicles

If undescended bilaterally, get chromosomal studies

Get MRI to identify testicle if you cannot feel it in inguinal canal

Tx: orchiopexy (inguinal incision)

If can't get testicle down → close, try again in 6 months

If won't come down again, divide spermatic vessels to get length

Adults w/ crypto-orchidism – resect testicle (almost certainly non-functional)

Varicoceles

Worry about **renal cell CA**

Left gonadal vein inserts into left renal vein

Obstruction by renal tumor causes varicocele

Increased infertility due to thrombosis/compression

Hydrocele in adult

If acute, need to suspect tumor elsewhere (possible retroperitoneum)

U/S will show that it is translucent

(see also pediatrics)

Testicular torsion

Involved testis usually not viable

Tx: bilateral orchiopexy (scrotal incision)

If testicle not viable, resection of the involved testicle and orchiopexy of contralateral testis

Bladder cancer

Transitional cell CA most common

Sx: **Painless hematuria** is classic

Tx:

T1 (muscle not involved)

Intra-vesicle BCG or;

Transurethral resection

T2 or greater (muscle wall invaded)

Cystectomy with ileal conduit

Chemotherapy (MVAC: methotrexate, vinblastine, Adriamycin, cisplatnin)

XRT

Metastatic DZ – chemotherapy

Ileal conduit standard after cystectomy

Avoids stasis and prevents the following:

Infection
Stones (Ca resorption)
Ureteral reflux

Surgery for kidney stones

Indications

Intractable pain

Recurrent infection

Progressive obstruction of ureter

Progressive renal damage (elevated creatnine)

Solitary kidney (risk of HD)

90% opaque

> 6 mm not going to pass easily

Tx: lithotripsy (best choice)

Other options:

Ureteroscopy w/ stone extraction or stent past obstruction

Percutaneous nephrostomy tube (just to relieve obstruction)

Open nephrolithotomy or urethotomy as a last resort

Gynecology

Ovarian cancer

Most common cause of gynecologic death

Decreased risk of ovarian cancer

> OCP's
> bilateral tubal ligation

Increased risk of ovarian cancer

> Nulliparity
> Late menopause
> Early menarche

Ovarian Tumors (3 basic types)

> **Epithelial Tumors** (Serous, endometrial, mucinous, clear cell, and borderline)
>
> > Most common type of ovarian tumor overall
> >
> > Most common type of ovarian tumor in post-menopausal women
> >
> > **Serous** most common sub-type
> >
> > **Clear cell** has the worst prognosis

> **Germ cell tumors**
>
> > Usually occur in pre-menopausal women
> >
> > **Teratoma** (dermoid cyst) most common subtype

> **Sex-cord stromal tumors**

Staging

I   Limited to one or both ovaries only

II   Limited just to the pelvis

III   Spread throughout the abdomen

IV   Distant metastatic spread

Bilateral ovary involvement - stage I

Debulking

Can be effective

Include omentectomy (improves chemo-XRT)

Tx: All stages get

TAH and BSO

Partial omentectomy

Selective para-aortic and pelvic lymphadenectomy

Also need:

Peritoneal washings

Bx from under right hemi-diaphragm

Bx of suspicious lesions

Washings from paracolic recess

Chemotherapy (cisplatnin and Taxol) and XRT post-op

Abortions

Missed

1st trimester vaginal bleeding

Closed os on pelvic exam

Gestational sac is seen on ultrasound, but no heartbeat

Threatened

1st trimester vaginal bleeding

Gestational sac is seen on ultrasound, and there is a heartbeat

Incomplete

Abortion tissue protrudes through os on exam

Ectopic

Presents with acute abdominal pain

beta-HCG is positive

Negative ultrasound for gestational sac

Patient has a history of a missed period, vaginal bleeding

Hypotension (this would be an emergency)

RF's previous tubal manipulation, PID, previous ectopic

MC location – ampullary portion of fallopian tubes

Surgical Emergency if the patient is hypotensive

Try to spare fallopian tube if possible

Mittelschmirtz

Rupture of graffian follicle cyst

Can be confused w/ appendicitis

14 days after the 1st day of menses

Tx: Appendectomy and close if found incidentally

Not sure if Graffian Follicle:

4 quadrant wash, send for cytology

Bx cyst wall (or mass if you're following the incidental mass pathway below)

Bx omentum

Look at all visceral surfaces for metastases, biopsy these areas, send to cytology

F/U w/ OB

Incidental ovarian cyst or mass at time of laparotomy

Follow the **Not sure if Graffian Follicle** pathway above

Do not perform oophrectomy unless you have an OB/GYN with you

Neurosurgery

Thoracic sympathectomy

Palmar and axillary hyperhidrosis – most take T2-T4 sympathetic nerves

MC complication – compensatory sweating in the lower extremities

Avoid taking T1 – can result in Horner's Syndrome (ptosis, miosis, and anhydrosis)

Nerve of Knutz

accessory nerve pathway between T1 and T2 that can result in refractory palmar sweating after sympathectomy

need to coagulate on bottom of the 2nd rib to divide the nerve of Knutz and avoid this complication

Orthopaedics

Upper extremity Injuries

Monteggia fracture

Fall with the elbow in partially flexed position

Proximal ulnar fracture

Radial head dislocation.

Tx: open reduction and internal fixation

Colles fracture

Fall on outstretched hand

Distal radius w/ possible ulnar styloid fracture

Tx: closed reduction usual

Galeazzi Fracture

Distal radial fracture

Radio-ulnar joint dislocation

Tx: **Children** – closed reduction

Adults - open reduction and internal fixation

Forearm fractures involving both the radius and ulna

    children – closed reduction

    adults – open reduction and internal fixation

Scaphoid fracture

    Snuffbox tenderness

    Can have negative x-ray

    Tx: all patients require cast to elbow, may need fixation

    Risk of **avascular necrosis**

Nursemaid's Elbow

    From pulling on an outstretched arm

    Radial head dislocation (at the elbow)

    Tx: closed reduction

Humeral Fracture

    Tx: usually treated with just a sling

Shoulder dislocation

    Tx: closed reduction

Forearm fasciotomy

Volar incision

Curvilinear (lazy S shape) so that all of the major nerves and
arteries are decompressed

Dorsal incision

Longitudinal incision (linear)

Need to open both the mobile extensor wad and extensor
digitorum communus muscle group compartments

<u>Indications for re-implantation after an amputation</u>:

Multiple digits

Thumb

Hand

Wrist

Forearm

At or proximal to elbow

Fingers in children

Individual digits distal to the insertion of the flexor digitorum superficialis on the middle phalynx

Child w/ tip of finger amputated – re-implant so nail bed can grow properly

Tx:

Place limb wrapped in plastic bag in ice-water container for transport to the facility

Abx's, wash off limb, tetanus shot

Re-implantation technique:

Tendon repair

4-0 Tevdek core suture 1 cm back on both ends of tendon
5-0 Tevdek interrupted sutures ½ cm back

Nerve repair – 10-0 prolenes just through epineurium

Vascular repair – 8-0 prolene

Place in cast for bones to heal

Supporative Tenosynovitis

Infectious spread along the flexor tendon sheaths

4 signs

Tenderness along the tendon sheath

Pain w/ passive motion of fingers

Swelling along the infected sheath

Semi-flexed position of the involved digit

Tx;

Elevation of affected limb

Splinting

Antibiotics

If prompt improvement does not occur → midaxial longitudinal incision and drainage

Rotator cuff tears

Muscle of the rotator cuff include:

supraspinatus

infraspinatus

teres minor

subscapularis

Acutely torn rotator cuff

Tx: sling and conservative tx

Surgical repair if patient requires a high level of activity or if the activities of daily living are affected

Paronychia

Infection underneath the nail bed

Painful

Tx: antibiotics and remove nail if purulent

Felon

Infection within terminal joint space on the finger

Tx: Incision along the medial and lateral aspects

Need to incise to prevent necrosis of tip of finger

Lower Extremity Injuries

Femoral shaft fracture

ORIF with intra-medullary rod

Femoral neck fracture

ORIF

Risk of avascular necrosis

Should not delay operation to avoid avascular necrosis

Posterior knee dislocation

All get angiogram to check for popliteal artery injury

Tibial plateau fracture and tibia-fibula fracture

ORIF

Nerve injured w/ lower extremity fasciotomy– common peroneal

Open fractures

These are considered infected – need washout

Place an external fixator

Pediatric Surgery

Hydrocoele

Usually have a persistent **processus vaginalis** (communicating) or this may have been obliterated (non-communicating)

Can be in **inguinal canal** or **scrotum**

U/S - will transluminate the hydrocoele if in scrotum (differentiates from a hernia)

Tx: Surgery at 1 year if not resolved or if it is felt to be a communicating hydrocoele (waxes and wanes in size)

Inguinal hernia

Persistent processus vaginalis

Varying degrees – can go all the way to the scrotum or stop short

Get U/S to make sure it's not a hydrocele (hydrocele will trans-illuminate)

Most common on the right

Tx: emergent operation if not able to reduce, o/w elective repair w/ **high ligation** (up to age 15 or so)

Consider 3 mm scope to look at the other side for hernia

Make sure testicle in scrotum at the end

Umbilical hernia

Failure of closure of linea alba

Usually close by age 3

Tx: surgery for

Failure to close by **age 5**

Incarcerated umbilical hernia

Patient has a **VP shunt**

Pyloric stenosis

Usually presents at 3–12 weeks

Projectile vomiting is classic

Can feel **a mass** in the RUQ (olive)

U/S – pylorus $\geq$ **4mm thick,** $\geq$ **14 mm long**

Projectile vomiting results in hypochloremic, hypokalemic metabolic alkalosis

Resuscitate (D_{10} ¼ NS w/ 10 mEq K) before OR

Tx: pyloromyotomy (try not to disrupt the mucosa)

Intussusception

Patients are usually 3 months to 3 years

Sx's: RUQ pain w/ sausage-like mass

Vomiting.

Currant jelly stools (from vascular congestion, this is <u>not</u> an indication for resection)

Abdominal distention

Occurs from invagination of one loop of intestine into another (often occurs at the level of the cecum)

Lead points in children

Enlarged Peyer's Patches (most common cause)

Meckel's diverticulum

Lymphoma

Approximately 15% have a recurrence after reduction (surgery if occurs again after 2nd time of reduction)

Tx: reduce with air-contrast enema

Approximately 80% successful (<u>no</u> surgery if reduced 1st time or with recurrence)

If it occurs a 3rd time, go to OR

Maximum pressure allowed with an **air-contrast enema is 120 mmHg**

Maximum column height allowed with a **barium enema** is **1 meter (3 feet)**

Should not go above these values because of the high perforation risk → go to OR

Do not pull on bowel to relieve, milk the intestine out

Diaphragmatic hernias

Survival 50%

Most common on **left** (80%)

Can have severe pulmonary hypertension of both lungs

Associated anomalies in 80% (cardiac, neural tube defects, malrotation)

Present at birth; usually in respiratory distress

CXR will show opacified chest on affected side (may see bowel loops)

Tx: High frequency ventilation

ECMO

Prostacyclin (pulmonary vasodilator)

Inhaled NO

Stabilize before OR - Abdominal approach, reduce bowel, repair defect ± mesh

Neuroblastoma

Most common solid abdominal malignancy in children

Most commonly presents as an asymptomatic mass

Other sx's:

>Secretory diarrhea

>Raccoon eyes (orbital metastases)

>**HTN**

>Opsomyoclonus syndrome (unsteady gait)

Most common location - **adrenals**

Usually see ↑ **catecholamines, VMA, HVA, and metanephrines**

Neural crest cells

AXR – can see calcifications

Worse prognosis - NSE, LDH, HVA, diploid tumors, and N-myc

Tx: resection (35% cured)

>If initially unresectable:

>>Give chemotherapy w/ cisplatnin and etoposide

>>Re-stage the patient

>>May be resectable after chemotherapy

Wilms tumor (nephroblastoma)

Most commonly presents as asymptomatic mass

   Other sx's: hematuria or HTN

10% bilateral

Prognosis - based on tumor grade

Worse prognosis – anaplastic, sarcomatous

Should resect pulmonary metastases if resectable

Tx: nephrectomy (90% cured)

   Venous extension in renal vein - the tumor can be extracted

   Avoid rupture of tumor which will increase the stage

   Bilateral tumors

      Pre-op chemo (vincristine and actinomycin)

      Partial kidney resection(s) to prevent need for dialysis

   If initially unresectable:

      Give chemotherapy w/ vincristine and actinomycin

      Re-stage the patient

      May be resectable after chemotherapy

   Pulmonary metastases – resect if resectable

   XRT for stages III and IV

Duodenal Atresia

Most common cause of duodenal obstruction in newborns (less than 1 week old)

Most commonly distal to ampulla of Vater (80%)

Can be associated with duodenal webs

Symptoms: **bilious vomiting,** feeding intolerance

Associated with polyhydramnios in mother

Associated anomalies include cardiac, renal and other GI anomalies

Down's syndrome in 20%

AXR - **double-bubble sign** (distended proximal duodenum and stomach)

Tx: fluid resuscitation

Can perform duodenoduodenostomy or duodeno-jejunostomy

Duodenal webs can cause persistent obstruction after repair

Malrotation

Bilious vomiting in a child < 2 indication for emergent UGI to look for malrotation

Ladd's bands

Extend out from the right retroperitoneum and cause duodenal obstruction

Volvulus

Compromises the superior mesenteric artery

Leads to infarction of the intestine

Results from failure of normal counter clockwise rotation (270°)

Dx: UGI

Duodenum does not cross the midline

May see obstruction

Tx: resect the Ladd's bands

Counterclockwise rotation

Place cecum in LLQ and secure it

Place duodenum in RUQ and secure it

Appendectomy (appendicitis would be on the wrong side of the abdomen and hard to diagnose in the future)

Duodenal webs can cause persistent bowel obstruction

Tracheoesophageal fistulas

Type C – most common (85%)

Proximal esophageal atresia (blind pouch)

Distal TEF

Sx's: newborn who **spits up feeds**

Excessive **drooling**

Aspiration w/ feeding

Difficulty placing NG tube into the stomach

VACTERL anomalies:

Vertebral

Anorectal (imperforate anus)

Cardiac

TE fistula

Radius/Renal anomalies

Limb anomalies

Tx: right thoracotomy

Perform primary repair

Bronch to locate fistula, find undiagnosed fistulas, assess for tracheomalacia

Circular myotomies – can be made in the proximal esophagus to get more length (1-3, each give 1 cm) – submucosa left intact (blood supply)

End to end anastomosis, absorbable suture; feeding tube through anastomosis

Can close up to **6 cm defects**

If primary repair not possible:

> **Distal esophagus is oversewn** and sutured to the pre-vertebral fascia

> Delayed primary repair after **daily proximal esophageal dilatations** for 1-2 months

> If that fails, esophageal **replacement w/ colon** may be necessary

Premature infants (< 2500 gm) or too ill for surgery → replogle tube, TPN (or G-tube), delayed repair

Most Common Complication after repair – GERD

Meconium ileus

Distal ileal obstruction from thickened meconium

Patients get abdominal distension, have vomiting

Sweat chloride test or PCR for Cl channel defect to look for cystic fibrosis

AXR: dilated loops of small bowel without air-fluid levels (meconium too thick to separate from bowel wall)

Tx: gastrograffin enema (N-acetylcysteine enema may be best) effective in 80%

OR if that does not relive the obstruction

Milk the obstruction out if requires OR

Hirschsprung's disease

Infants failing to pass meconium in 1st 24 hours suggests disease

Patients get abdominal distension, which can lead to colitis in some

Explosive release of watery stool w/ anorectal exam classic finding but this is not diagnostic

Rectal biopsy – is the diagnostic procedure of choice

Shows absence of ganglion cells in the myenteric plexus

Tx: Resect colon proximal to level of ganglion cells

Connect colon to anus (Soave or Duhamel)

May need interim colostomy before hooking up to anus

Printed in the United States
125432LV00002B/96/A

9 781427 602527